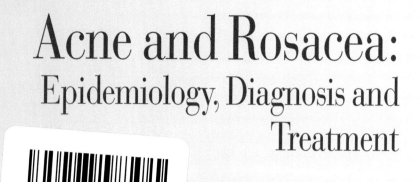

Acne and Rosacea:
Epidemiology, Diagnosis and Treatment

T0248635

David J. Goldberg, MD, JD

Clinical Professor of Dermatology & Director of Laser Research,

Mount Sinai School of Medicine,

New York, NY

Clinical Professor of Dermatology & Chief of Dermatologic Surgery

UMDNJ New Jersey Medical School,

Newark, NJ

Adjunct Professor of Law

Fordham Law School,

New York, NY

Director, Skin Laser & Surgery Specialists,

New York, NY

Alexander L. Berlin, MD

Clinical Assistant Professor of Dermatology,

UMDNJ New Jersey Medical School,

Newark, NJ

Director of Mohs & Cosmetic Surgery,

US Dermatology Medical Group - Mullanax Dermatology Associates

Arlington, TX.

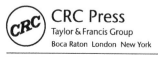

CRC Press
Taylor & Francis Group
Boca Raton London New York

CRC Press is an imprint of the
Taylor & Francis Group, an **informa** business

CRC Press
Taylor & Francis Group
6000 Broken Sound Parkway NW, Suite 300
Boca Raton, FL 33487-2742

© 2012 by Taylor & Francis Group, LLC
CRC Press is an imprint of Taylor & Francis Group, an Informa business

First issued in paperback 2019

No claim to original U.S. Government works

ISBN 13: 978-0-367-45221-6 (pbk)
ISBN 13: 978-1-84076-150-4 (hbk)

Visit the Taylor & Francis Web site at
http://www.taylorandfrancis.com

and the CRC Press Web site at
http://www.crcpress.com

CONTENTS

ABBREVIATIONS

ALA	aminolevulinic acid	MMP	matrix metal loproteinase
AP	activator protein	MTZ	microscopic treatment zone
CAP	cationic antimicrobial protein	Nd:YAG	neodymium:yttrium–aluminum–garnet
CRABP	cytosolic retinoic acid-binding protein	PABA	para-aminobenzoic acid
CROSS	chemical reconstruction of skin scars	PDL	pulsed-dye laser
DHEA-S	dehydroepiandrosterone sulfate	PDT	photodynamic therapy
DHT	dihydrotestosterone	Pp	protoporphyrin
DISH	diffuse idiopathic skeletal hyperostosis	PP	papulopustular (rosacea)
Er:YAG	erbium:yttrium–aluminum–garnet (laser)	RAR	retinoic acid receptor
Er:YSGG	erbium:yttrium–scandium–gallium-garnet (laser)	RARE	retinoic acid response element
		RF	radiofrequency
ET	erythematotelangiectatic (rosacea)	ROS	reactive oxygen species
FDA	Food and Drug Administration	RXR	retinoid X receptor
G6PD	glucose-6-phosphate dehydrogenase	SCTE	stratum corneum tryptic enzyme
HIV	human immunodeficiency virus	TCA	trichloroacetic acid
ICAM	intercellular adhesion molecule	TLR	Toll-like receptor
IGF	insulin-like growth factor	TNF	tumor necrosis factor
IL	interleukin	TRT	thermal relaxation time
IPL	intense pulsed light	UV	ultraviolet
KTP	potassium titanyl phosphate (laser)	VEGF	vascular endothelial growth factor
LED	light-emitting diode		
MAL	methyl aminolevulinate		

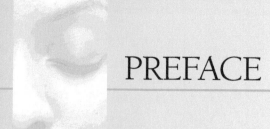

PREFACE

Acne and rosacea are two incredibly common skin problems that have both a medical and cosmetic impact on the daily lives of millions of people. Much has been written in books and journal articles about the medical treatment of acne and rosacea. Similarly, much has been written in books and journal articles about the cosmetic treatment of acne and rosacea. This book is unique in that it presents an objective look at both the medical and cosmetic treatments of these two skin disorders.

The first four chapters deal with acne and acne scars and the medical and laser/light treatments used to treat patients with these problems. The next three chapters take the same approach to rosacea. Finally, the last chapter discusses the treatment of sebaceous hyperplasia.

We greatly appreciate the information provided by Professor Anthony Chu of Hammersmith Hospital, London, UK, on the availability of various therapeutic agents outside of the US.

David J. Goldberg
Alexander L. Berlin

New York, NY
and Arlington, TX

Disclaimer
The advice and information given in this book are believed to be true and accurate at the time of going to press. However, not all drugs, formulations, and devices are currently available in all countries, and readers are advised to check local availability and prescribing regimens.

1 ACNE VULGARIS – EPIDEMIOLOGY AND PATHOPHYSIOLOGY

INTRODUCTION

ACNE vulgaris is a common disorder of the pilosebaceous unit affecting millions of people worldwide. Although most frequently encountered in adolescents, acne may persist well into adulthood and lead to significant physical and psychological impairment in those affected. The severity of acne may vary significantly from the mildest comedonal forms (**1**) to a severe and debilitating condition (**2**). In addition to the face, the chest, back, and shoulders are also commonly affected (**3, 4**).

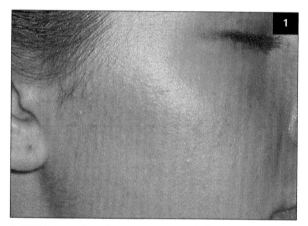

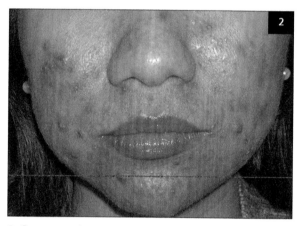

1 Mild comedonal acne on a patient's face.

2 Severe cystic acne.

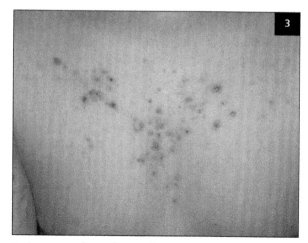

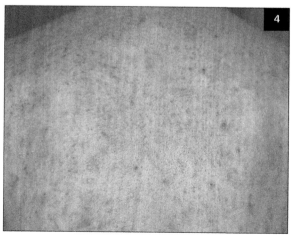

3 Acne papules and **pustules** on the chest.

4 Acne papules associated with extensive postinflammatory hyperpigmentation on a patient's back.

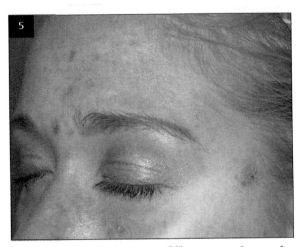

5 In acné excoriée des jeunes filles, patients frequently manipulate their acne lesions, leading to prolonged healing time and often, scarring.

Numerous factors, both intrinsic and extrinsic (5), may underlie the development and the progression of the disease.

EPIDEMIOLOGY

Acne is the most common cutaneous disorder in the Western world. In the United States, its prevalence has been variably estimated at between 17 and 45 million people (Berson *et al.* 2003; White 1998). This number is typically based on a landmark publication by Kraning & Odland (1979), which estimated the prevalence of acne in persons aged 12–24 years at 85%.

Several studies have documented that a significant portion of acne sufferers are postadolescent or adult (Collier *et al.* 2008; Cunliffe & Gould 1979; Goulden *et al.* 1997; Poli *et al.* 2001, Stern 1992).A recent study based on 1013 surveys found the overall prevalence of acne in patients 20 years of age and older to be 73.3% (Collier et al. 2008). Among such patients, women are affected at higher rates than men in all age categories. Thus, more recent studies place the incidence of clinically-important adult acne at 12% of women and 3% of men over 25 years of age. If milder, 'physiologic' acne is taken into consideration, the prevalence increases to 54% of women and 40% of men (Goulden *et al.* 1997). Adult acne may present as a continuation of the teenage disease process or may arise *de novo*. Acne is also encountered in the preadolescent population, including neonates and, less commonly, infants and preteens (Cunliffe *et al.* 2001; Jansen *et al.* 1997; Lucky 1998).

The prevalence of acne in individuals with skin of color has, likewise, been investigated in several studies (**6, 7**). Thus, Halder *et al.* (1983) reported acne being present in 27.7% of the Black patients and 29.5% of the Caucasian patients. Additional studies of adult patients in the United Kingdom and Singapore have placed the prevalence of adult acne at 13.7% of the Black patients and 10.9% of the Indian and Asian patients (Child *et al.* 1999; Goh & Akarapanth 1994). It has also been shown that the presence of significant inflammation, resulting in the clinical appearance of nodulocystic acne, is more common in Caucasian and Hispanic patients than in their Black counterparts (Wilkins & Voorhees 1970). More recent evidence indicates that subclinical, microscopic inflammation may be more common in the latter group (Halder *et al.* 1996).

It has also been suggested that certain non-westernized societies demonstrate significantly lower prevalence of acne (Cordain *et al.* 2002; Schaefer 1971; Steiner 1946). The cause of such disparity is unclear and although nutritional factors have been suggested as the cause of lower acne rates, this inference has so far not been conclusively substantiated (Bershad 2003).

The issue of nutrition and its influence, or lack thereof, on acne has long been a highly contested one (Adebamowo *et al.* 2005; Bershad 2003; Bershad 2005; Cordain 2005; Danby 2005; Kaymak *et al.* 2007; Logan 2003; Smith *et al.* 2007; Treloar 2003). Proponents of the link between acne and nutrition frequently cite nutritional influence on serum hormone levels, such as insulin-like growth factor (IGF)-1 and IGF binding protein-3, to demonstrate the purported effect on acne. Thus, foods with a low glycemic load–those that cause least elevation of blood glucose and have lowest carbohydrate content–as well as diets high in omega-3 essential fatty acids, have been advocated as beneficial for acne patients (Cordain 2005; Logan 2003; Smith *et al.* 2007; Treloar *et al.* 2008). Additionally, milk has been proposed as a potential culprit in acne causation, with arguments being raised as to the presence of various hormones in the consumed product (Adebamowo *et al.* 2005, Danby 2005). On the other hand, those refuting the link between acne and nutrition may cite two flawed studies from over 30 years ago (Anderson 1971; Fulton *et al.* 1969). In reality, controlling diet in a study is difficult, especially when it involves teenagers. As it stands now, there are far too few

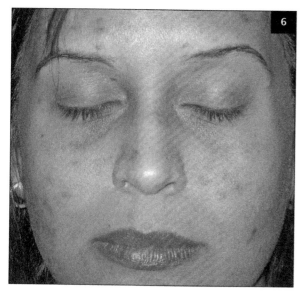

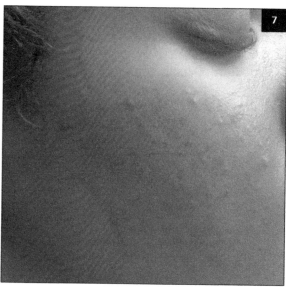

6 **Postinflammatory hyperpigmentation** is a common consequence of acne in patients with darker skin tones, such as this Indian patient.

7 **Extensive postinflammatory hyperpigmentation** in an African-American patient with acne.

large, well-designed, well-controlled prospective clinical studies to substantiate either point of view. This is in accordance with the current guidelines of care from the American Academy of Dermatology (Strauss *et al.* 2007).

Smoking and its influence on acne prevalence and severity has been investigated in several published clinical trials (Chuh *et al.* 2004; Firooz *et al.* 2005; Jemec *et al.* 2002; Klaz *et al.* 2006; Mills *et al.* 1993; Rombouts *et al.* 2007; Schafer *et al.* 2001). Of these studies, two suggested a positive association between smoking and acne, three proposed a negative one, and two found no association. Thus, the evidence so far is inconclusive; however, taking into consideration other, more serious health risks associated with smoking, cessation should always be encouraged.

Very importantly, acne may arise in a number of genetic and endocrinologic conditions, and the genetic component of acne vulgaris has been well documented. For example, patients with the XYY genotype and those with polycystic ovarian syndrome, hyperandrogenism, and elevated serum cortisol levels have a significantly increased risk of developing acne (Lowenstein 2006; Mann *et al.* 2007; New & Wilson 1999; Stratakis *et al.* 1998; The Rotterdam ESHRE/ASRM-Sponsored PCOS consensus workshop group 2004; Voorhees *et al.* 1972)

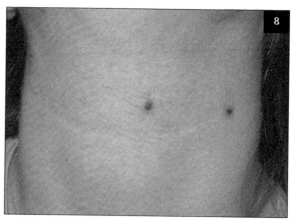

8 **A combination of acne and hirsutism,** such as on the neck of this patient, may point to an underlying state of hyperandrogenism.

(8). Additionally, there is a high level of concordance in acne severity between monozygotic twins, while adult acne has been demonstrated to occur with a much higher frequency in those with first-degree relatives suffering from the same condition (Bataille *et al.* 2002; Evans *et al.* 2005; Friedman 1984; Goulden *et al.* 1999; Lee & Cooper 2006).

CLINICAL ASSESSMENT OF ACNE VULGARIS

Acne vulgaris frequently presents with a combination of morphological features, including open and closed comedones, papules, pustules, and nodules (**9–11**). The mildest form of acne is comedonal acne, characterized by the absence of inflammatory lesions. On the other side of the spectrum is acne conglobata, presenting with large, interconnecting, tender abscesses and irregular scars causing profound disfigurement. More acute and severe in presentation is acne fulminans, a multisystem syndrome of sudden onset, characterized by necrotizing acne abscesses associated with fever, lytic bone lesions, polyarthritis, and laboratory abnormalities (Jansen & Plewig 1998; Seukeran & Cunliffe 1999).

In order to assess the initial severity of acne and to follow patient progress in a clinical setting, as well as to be able to evaluate the efficacy of various therapeutic agents in clinical trials, an objective measurement technique is important. Numerous systems have been developed over the years; however, no clear winner has so far emerged.

The first published attempt to measure the severity of disease in acne appeared in a dermatological textbook in 1956 (Pillsbury *et al.* 1956). This technique assigned grades to acne severity, ranging from 1 to 4, based on the overall type and number of lesions, the predominant lesion, and the extent of involvement. Several modified

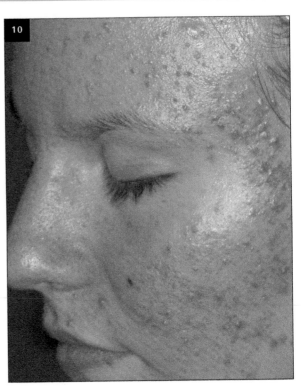

10 **Extensive acne papules** on a patient's face.

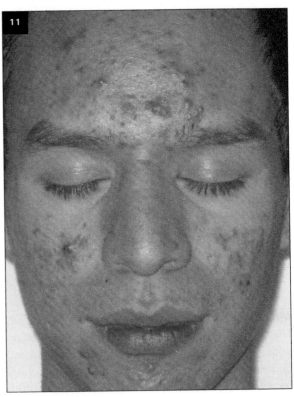

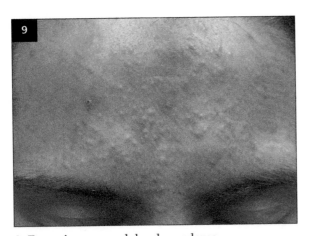

9 **Extensive open** and closed comedones.

11 **Nodulocystic acne.**

grading systems have since been introduced, some utilizing reference photographs or polarized light photography (Burke & Cunliffe 1984; Cook *et al.* 1979; Doshi *et al.* 1997; James & Tisserand 1958; Phillips *et al.* 1997).

Developing in parallel with acne grading techniques were the various systems emphasizing lesion counts (Christiansen *et al.* 1976; Lucky *et al.* 1996; Michaelson *et al.* 1977; Witkowski & Simons 1966). This method typically involves counting individual lesions in each morphological category and frequently subdivides the face into separate regions. Lesion counting was recently validated and appears to be more objective than acne grading (Lucky *et al.* 1996). Still, multiple arguments between acne graders and lesion counters have arisen in the literature (Shalita *et al.* 1997; Witkowski & Parish 1999), and none of the current methods of acne assessment are entirely perfect. Some systems actually combine lesion counting with overall grading (Plewig & Kligman 1975). In reality, two standardized, validated systems are likely necessary: one that can be easily and rapidly applied in a clinical setting without the need for intricate instrumentation, and a separate, more sensitive approach that can be utilized in clinical research.

PATHOPHYSIOLOGY OF ACNE VULGARIS

Over the last several years, our understanding of the pathogenesis of acne has increased dramatically. The new research findings will likely lead to new advances in acne therapy, as well as the elucidation of pathogenesis of other cutaneous conditions.

The traditional view of the pathogenesis of acne is frequently termed the microcomedone theory. According to this theory, the initial step in the disease process is hyperkeratosis of the follicular lining in the proximal part of the upper portion of the follicle, the infrainfundibulum. This is accompanied by the increased cohesiveness of the corneocytes within this lining and results in a bottleneck effect within the follicle. As the shed keratinocytes and sebum continue to accumulate, they undergo a transformation into whorled lamellar concretions, resulting in a clinical appearance of a comedone. *Propionibacterium acnes* (*P. acnes*) bacteria proliferate within an expanding comedone, prompt a host response, and contribute to the production of inflammatory acne, clinically manifesting as papules and pustules. Finally, as the shed

keratinocytes and sebum continue to accumulate, internal pressure leads to the rupture of the comedo wall with subsequent marked inflammation and nodule formation. Such intense inflammation may eventually lead to scarring (**12**).

Although the basic tenets of the theory still appear to be valid, new research findings shed more light on the specific pathogenetic mechanisms underlying the various stages of the disease process and the progression from one stage to another. Additionally, the order of these events has been challenged by the new findings, suggesting a more complicated interplay of the various factors contributing to the condition. Some of these newer findings will now be examined.

Follicular hyperkeratinization and corneocyte cohesiveness

Although considered key to the process of comedone formation, the process of follicular hyperkeratinization is incompletely understood. Using staining for Ki-67 antigen, it has been demonstrated that cellular

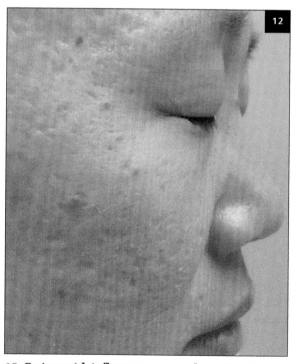

12 Patient with inflammatory papules and resultant acne scars.

proliferation within comedones, as well as within normal follicles in acne-affected sites, is higher than that in normal follicles in unaffected skin (Knaggs et al. 1994a). It has also been shown that the addition of interleukin (IL)-1 alpha to the infrainfundibular segment causes hypercornification (Guy et al. 1996). Alternatively, it has been suggested that locally reduced sebum levels of linoleic acid, an essential fatty acid, may induce hyperkeratosis in the affected follicles (Downing et al. 1986).

An analysis of the desmosomal components, however, failed to demonstrate a difference between acne follicles and normal controls, suggesting that the increased cohesiveness of the corneocytes within comedones is not due to alterations in these linking proteins (Knaggs et al. 1994b). Recently, it has been suggested that the increased adhesion of corneocytes within comedones is actually due to a glue-like biofilm produced by the P. acnes bacteria (Burkhart & Burkhart 2007). A biofilm is an aggregate of microorganisms enveloped in an extracellular polysaccharide lining. Although the formation of the P. acnes biofilm has been shown (Burkhart & Burkhart 2006), its actual role in the increased adhesiveness of the follicular corneocytes has yet to be demonstrated. This finding may, however, challenge the traditionally-established order of events in the pathophysiology of acne.

Sebum production and hormonal influences

Androgens have long been implicated in the pathogenesis of acne. Androgens appear to play an essential role in regulating sebum production. Thus, acne development and sebaceous gland activity in prepubertal boys and girls correlate with elevated serum levels of dehydroepiandrosterone sulfate (DHEA-S) (Lucky et al. 1994; Stewart et al. 1992). This hormone is mainly produced in the adrenal glands, and its elevation in prepubertal children heralds the onset of adrenarche. As well, androgen-insensitive individuals do not produce sebum and are not affected by acne (Imperato-McGinley et al. 1993). Finally, a correlation between severe (but not necessarily mild or moderate) acne and elevated serum androgens has been demonstrated (Aizawa et al. 1995; Lucky et al. 1983; Marynick et al. 1983).

Androgens are generated from the cholesterol molecule (13). The reader is encouraged to review this steroidogenic pathway, which was recently summarized in detail by Chen et al. (2002). It has now also been shown that, in addition to the gonads and the adrenal glands, this process takes place in the epidermis and in sebaceous glands (Menon et al. 1985; Smythe et al. 1998); however, the relative contribution of each of these sources is unknown.

Once synthesized, testosterone is converted to dihydrotestosterone (DHT) through the action of 5alpha-reductase. Type 1 isozyme has been shown to be most active in the sebaceous glands (Fritsch et al. 2001), whereas type 2 is most prominent in the prostate gland. It has been shown that the activity of 5alpha-reductase is greater in acne-prone locations, such as the face, compared to nonacne-prone skin (Thiboutot et al. 1995). Testosterone and DHT are the major androgens that interact with the androgen receptors in sebaceous glands, although DHT is 5–10 times more potent in this interaction. Once bound, the androgen–receptor complex appears to regulate the expression of genes responsible for cellular growth and sebum production within sebocytes. However, the exact mechanism of this interaction has not yet been completely elucidated.

The role of estrogens in acne is uncertain. Although it has been shown that very large doses of exogenous estrogen are able to suppress sebum production (Strauss & Pochi 1964), it is unclear what function (if any) the physiologic levels of estrogens play in the regulation of the sebaceous glands. Estradiol and the less potent estrone can be derived from testosterone through the actions of aromatase and 17beta-hydroxysteroid dehydrogenase. Both of these enzymes are present in the skin, as well as other peripheral tissues (Sawaya & Price 1997). The exact role of these hormones in acne will have to be established in future studies.

Insulin-like growth factor-1 (IGF-1), a hormone closely related to the human growth hormone, has recently been investigated as a possible contributing factor to the development of acne. IGF-1 levels have been found to be significantly elevated in postadolescent women with acne (Aizawa & Niimura 1995) and to be correlated with the number of clinical acne lesions in women, but not in men (Cappel et al. 2005). Although these studies suggest that IGF-1 may directly contribute to the etiology of acne, the complex nature of interdependence of various hormones in the skin is not completely understood and deserves further studying. Additionally, receptors for other hormones,

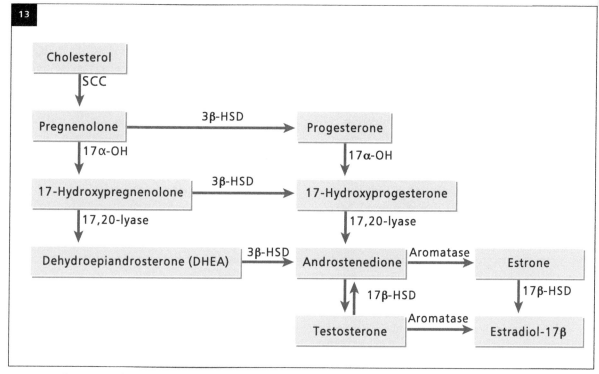

13 Steroidogenic pathway. SCC: side chain cleavage; 3β -HSD: 3β-hydroxysteroid dehydrogenase; 17α-OH: 17α hydroylase; 17β-HSD: 17β-hydroxysteroid dehydrogenase.

including melanocortin-5, corticotrophin-releasing hormone, and others, have also been demonstrated in human sebaceous glands (Thiboutot *et al*. 2000; Zouboulis *et al*. 2002). Although their exact role in the onset and propagation of acne is currently unknown, it has been suggested that these neuroendocrine mediators may underlie the effect of stress on acne (Zouboulis & Bohm 2004).

Role of *Propionibacterium acnes* and the host immune system

P. acnes is a weakly Gram-positive, non-motile, rod-shaped coryneform or diphtheroid anerobic bacterium long implicated in the pathogenesis of acne. In fact, several studies have demonstrated a higher number of *P. acnes* bacteria on the skin of children and teenagers with acne compared to age-matched controls without acne (Leyden *et al*. 1975; Leyden *et al*. 1998; Mourelatos *et al*. 2007). *P. acnes* is known to produce porphyrins, particularly coproporphyrin III, which fluoresces under Wood's light. *P. acnes* also synthesizes

phosphatidyl inositol, akin to eukaryotes, and has a distinctive structure of peptidoglycans in the cell wall (Kamisango *et al*. 1982). In addition, *P. acnes* produces various proteases, hyaluronidases, and lipases, which contribute to tissue injury (Hoeffler 1977; Ingham *et al*. 1980; Ingham *et al*. 1981; Puhvel & Reisner 1972). These properties appear to contribute to the complex interaction between the bacterium and the host immune system, the details of which are now emerging from the latest research.

Several proinflammatory cytokines, including tumor necrosis factor (TNF)-alpha, IL-1 beta, and IL-8, have previously been shown to be induced by *P. acnes* (Nagy *et al*. 2005; Schaller *et al*. 2005; Vowels *et al*. 1995). IL-8 may be of particular importance in the host inflammatory response, as it is a major chemotactic factor for neutrophils. In addition, *P. acnes* has been shown to induce the expression of human beta-defensin 4 (previously known as beta-defensin 2), an antimicrobial peptide (Nagy *et al*. 2005). More recently, cDNA microarray technology allowed simultaneous examination of multiple genes. Thus, a recent study by Trivedi *et al.* (2006) demonstrated upregulation in a variety of additional genes involved in inflammation and apoptosis, such as granzyme B, responsible for cell lysis in cell-mediated immune response.

Moreover, an elevation in activator protein (AP)-1, a transcription factor involved in inflammation, was recently demonstrated in acne lesions by Kang *et al.* (2005). Among the various genes regulated by AP-1 are several matrix metalloproteinases (MMPs), which are directly responsible for extracellular matrix degradation. Indeed, the levels of MMP-1 (collagenase-1), MMP-3 (stromelysin 1), MMP-8 (neutrophil collagenase or collagenase-2), and MMP-9 (gelatinase or collagenase-4) have been shown to be significantly elevated in inflammatory acne (Kang *et al.* 2005; Trivedi *et al.* 2006).

With the pioneering work by Kim *et al.* (2002), these research findings now appear to be linked. *P. acnes* has now been shown to activate Toll-like receptor (TLR)-2. TLRs are transmembrane receptors that mediate the immune response to molecular patterns conserved among microorganisms. TLRs are expressed on the cells of the innate immune system, including monocytes, macrophages, dendritic cells, and neutrophils. Some TLRs also appear to be constitutively or inducibly expressed on keratinocytes (Baker *et al.* 2003; Pivarcsi *et al.* 2003). In acne lesions, expression of TLR-2, which recognizes peptidoglycans from Gram-positive bacteria, has been demonstrated on macrophages in the perifollicular regions (Kim *et al.* 2002).

When activated, TLR-2 triggers a MyD88-dependent pathway that results in the nuclear translocation of NF-kappaB, a transcription factor. NF-kappaB then modulates the expression of various inflammatory cytokines and chemokines (Takeda & Akira 2004), most notably TNF-alpha and IL-1 beta, as well as several antimicrobial peptides (Nagy *et al.* 2005). TNF-alpha and IL-1 beta may then act in an autocrine or paracrine manner to stimulate further immune response. Additionally, they can induce the activation of AP-1 (Whitmarsh & Davis 1996), thus leading to the expression of MMPs, as described above. Of interest, the induction of IL-12 production by monocytes, which promotes the development of Th1-mediated immune responses, was also demonstrated to occur through the activation of TLR-2 by *P. acnes* (Kim *et al.* 2002), thus linking the innate and the acquired immune systems.

As the intricacies of the immune system and the host–pathogen interaction are further elucidated, additional factors underlying the initiation and the propagation of the pathological processes in acne will likely be discovered. This will be crucial to the development of new strategies in the prevention and treatment of this common condition.

2 ACNE VULGARIS – CURRENT MEDICAL THERAPEUTICS

INTRODUCTION

NUMEROUS therapeutic agents have been developed over the years for the treatment of acne vulgaris (*Table 1*). Although the mechanism of action of some of these agents has not been completely elucidated, most affect one or more of the etiological factors in acne. As research into the pathophysiology of this common disorder continues, additional, more effective therapeutic modalities will likely become available in the years to come.

This chapter will present current information on the most commonly utilized medical treatments. Although additional therapeutic agents have been tried in this condition, sufficient data from randomized prospective studies are lacking or incomplete, and some agents are not yet available in the US; thus, these agents will be beyond the scope of this chapter.

TOPICAL AGENTS

Topical agents are the mainstay of acne therapy. They are frequently used alone in mild cases, but are frequently combined with the oral agents in moderate to severe acne or in resistant cases.

Although most topical agents are left on the surface of the skin, some, such as cleansers, washes, and masks, are removed after only a short contact, thus lessening their absorption and, possibly, adverse effects.

Benzoyl peroxide

Benzoyl peroxide has been available both by prescription and over-the-counter for over 50 years, making it one of the most commonly used medications in acne. It is also available in several commercially-available combinations with topical antibacterial agents, to be covered later in this chapter. Numerous formulations are now available, with concentrations ranging from 2.5% to 10%, and may be used once or twice daily, depending on tolerability and the use of other topical agents. Newer formulations include

microspheres (currently only available in the US) to slow the delivery of the active ingredient and to reduce its irritant potential, and a micronized form thought to improve follicular penetration (Del Rosso 2008).

Benzoyl peroxide seems to have bactericidal, keratolytic, and comedolytic properties (Cunliffe *et al.* 1983; Waller *et al.* 2006). Its antibacterial properties are

Topical	Benzoyl peroxide
	Antibiotics
	Clindamycin
	Erythromycin
	Retinoids
	Adapalene
	Tretinoin
	Tazarotene
	Isotretinoin*
	Azelaic acid
	Sulfur
	Sodium sulfacetamide
Oral	Antibiotics
	Tetracyclines
	Azithromycin
	Trimethoprim +/- sulfamethoxazole
	Isotretinoin
	Hormonal agents
	Spironolactone
	Oral contraceptive agents

*not available in the US.

Table 1 Agents commonly used in the treatment of acne vulgaris

thought to derive from the generation of free-radical oxygen species. In randomized, prospective comparison studies, benzoyl peroxide has been found to be at least as effective in its bactericidal action as topical clindamycin or erythromycin (Burke *et al.* 1983; Swinyer *et al.* 1988).

No serious adverse effects of benzoyl peroxide have been reported. The most common side-effects include dryness, peeling, and erythema. As well, allergic contact dermatitis may develop in up to 2.5% of patients (Morelli *et al.* 1989). Patients should also be cautioned about the bleaching action of benzoyl peroxide to avoid ruining their clothes and towels.

Although no interactions between benzoyl peroxide and systemic agents have been reported, it is important to note that topical tretinoin, but not the newer retinoids adapalene and tazarotene, may be inactivated when applied concurrently with benzoyl peroxide (Martin *et al.* 1998; Shroot 1998). Benzoyl peroxide is a Food and Drug Administration (FDA) pregnancy category C agent and should, therefore, only be used in this population when clearly required. Its excretion in breast milk has not been studied.

Antibiotics

In the US, clindamycin and erythromycin are two topical antibiotic agents indicated for the treatment of acne vulgaris. Both are available in numerous formulations containing 1% clindamycin phosphate or 2–3% erythromycin, as well as several combination products with benzoyl peroxide and, in the case of clindamycin, with topical retinoids. In addition, a combined erythromycin–isotretinoin gel is available outside the US. Both clindamycin and erythromycin are typically used once to twice daily.

Clindamycin belongs to a lincosamide family of antibacterial agents. Its mechanism of action is direct attachment to the 50S subunit of the bacterial ribosome and subsequent inhibition of bacterial protein synthesis (Sadick 2007). Some studies have documented detectable urine, but not serum, concentrations of metabolites following proper topical application of clindamycin hydrochloride (Barza *et al.* 1982; Thomsen *et al.* 1980). No detectable urine levels have been documented with clindamycin phosphate (Stoughton *et al.* 1980). However, although low, the systemic bioavailability of topically-applied clindamycin should be taken into consideration, especially if large surfaces are being treated.

Adverse effects of orally-administered clindamycin may include granulocytopenia, hepatotoxicity, diarrhea, and pseudomembranous colitis (Aygun *et al.* 2007; Bubalo *et al.* 2003; Mylonakis *et al.* 2001; Pisciotta 1993). Of these, only the latter two have been documented following topical application of clindamycin and directly attributed to the medication (Becker *et al.* 1981; Milstone *et al.* 1981, Parry & Rha 1986). Pseudomembranous colitis, a serious and potentially life-threatening condition, results from the intestinal overgrowth of toxin-producing *Clostridium difficile*. Thus, topical clindamycin is contraindicated in patients with history of pseudomembranous colitis or inflammatory bowel disease.

The more commonly encountered and less serious adverse effects of topical clindamycin include erythema and scaling at the application site; these are more frequent with clindamycin solution than with either the gel or the lotion formulations (Goltz *et al.* 1985; Parker 1987). Although oral clindamycin potentiates the action of neuromuscular blockers, no such interaction has ever been documented with the topical agent, likely due to nearly negligible systemic absorption. Of potential clinical relevance, clindamycin and erythromycin have been found to be antagonistic *in vitro*; thus, concurrent use should be avoided (Igarashi *et al.* 1969). Topical clindamycin is an FDA pregnancy category B agent. Although orally-administered clindamycin is excreted in breast milk, no adverse effects in infants have been documented with the topical application.

Erythromycin belongs to the macrolide family of antibacterials. It reversibly binds the 50S subunit of the bacterial ribosome, thus inhibiting protein synthesis (Sadick 2007). Following topical application, systemic absorption appears to be very low, with no detectable serum levels (Schmidt *et al.* 1983).

Although common adverse effects of oral erythromycin may include abdominal cramps, nausea, vomiting, hepatitis, cholestasis, ototoxicity, and hypersensitivity reactions (Jorro *et al.* 1996; Keeffe *et al.* 1982; McGhan & Merchant 2003), these have not been reported with the topical formulations. Application-site adverse effects may include pruritus, burning, erythema, and peeling. Oral, but not topical, erythromycin has been found to prolong QT interval when combined with several other medications, no longer available on the market in the US, including cisapride, astemizole, and terfenadine. Topical erythromycin is an FDA pregnancy category B agent. Although oral erythromycin is known to be excreted in breast milk, such occurrence has not been documented with the topical formulations. However, because of a possible link between erythromycin use during lactation in the first weeks of life and the development of hypertrophic pyloric stenosis, caution should be exercised in this population (Maheshwai 2007).

Although both agents have been documented as efficacious in numerous studies, a recent meta-analysis of clinical trials of clindamycin and erythromycin used as monotherapy for acne revealed a two- to threefold decrease in the efficacy of erythromycin from the 1970s to 1990s (Simonart & Dramaix 2005). No similar findings were noted in the case of clindamycin. This suggests the emergence and propagation of erythromycin-resistant *P. acnes* bacteria. The previously mentioned combinations of topical antibacterial agents and benzoyl peroxide appear to be more efficacious in the treatment of inflammatory lesions and at reducing *P. acnes* counts, and are associated with significantly lower rates of bacterial resistance (Leyden *et al.* 2001a, b; Lookingbill *et al.* 1997). For these reasons, implementation of combination therapy utilizing benzoyl peroxide from the outset, rather than antibacterial monotherapy, is advocated by numerous authors.

Retinoids

Because of their chemical similarity to vitamin A (retinol), topical agents in this category were originally termed retinoids. With the discovery of retinoic acid receptors (RARS) and retinoid X receptors (RXR), the term came to be applied to chemical compounds that activate these receptors (Mangelsdorf *et al.* 1990; Petkovich *et al.* 1987). Three agents are currently FDA-approved in the US for the treatment of acne vulgaris. These include a first-generation retinoid tretinoin (all-*trans* retinoic acid), and second-generation retinoids adapalene (an aromatic naphthoic acid derivative) and tazarotene (an acetylenic retinoid). Topical isotretinoin, by itself and with erythromycin, is also available outside the US.

Numerous formulations of retinoids are currently on the market with differing availability throughout the world. Topical tretinoin is available in cream, solution (with 4% erythromycin outside the US), or gel forms ranging in concentration from 0.01% to 0.1%, as well as

the somewhat less irritating microsphere and delayed-release gel formulations. Adapalene is currently available as a 0.1% cream, solution, or gel, and, most recently, as a 0.3% gel. Tazarotene formulations include 0.05% cream and gel and 0.1% cream and gel, although only the latter two are FDA-approved for the treatment of acne. Outside the US, topical isotretinoin is available as a 0.05% gel. In addition, a combination gel that contains topical tretinoin 0.025% and clindamycin 1.2% is now available in the US, whereas a combination of topical adapalene 0.1% and benzoyl peroxide 2.5% is currently only available outside the US. Because of the photolabile nature of tretinoin, it is usually used at nighttime. Although adapalene and tazarotene are stable under light and oxidative conditions, they are most commonly also used at night to decrease local irritation and the risk of sunburn (Shroot 1998).

The mechanism of action of topical retinoids in acne is not completely understood, but appears to involve the inhibition of corneocyte proliferation and hyperkeratinization in the follicle, comedolysis, and inhibition of inflammation (Lavker *et al.* 1992; Liu *et al.* 2005; Marcelo & Madison 1984; Mills & Kligman 1983; Monzon *et al.* 1996; Presland *et al.* 2001; Tenaud *et al.* 2007).

As previously mentioned, retinoids bind and activate RAR or RXR nuclear receptors. These receptors are homologous to human glucocorticoid, vitamin D_3, and thyroid hormone receptors, but have significantly different ligand-binding domains (Mangelsdorf *et al.* 1990). To date, three subtypes (α, β, and γ) and isoforms of each of the RAR and RXR have been identified. Tretinoin binds to all subtypes of RAR and, following isomerization to 9-*cis* retinoic acid, can also bind and activate the RXRs. On the other hand, adapalene and tazarotenic acid, the active metabolite of tazarotene, preferentially bind RAR-β and -γ, but not RAR-α or the RXR subtypes (Chandraratna 1996; Shroot 1998). Once activated, RAR may form a heterodimer with RXR; alternatively, RXR may also form a homodimer. Retinoid receptor dimers then bind to specific DNA regulatory sequences, also known as retinoic acid response elements (RAREs). This binding appears to regulate directly the transcription of genes involved in normalization of keratinization and cellular adhesion; however, the full details of this complex process have not yet been elucidated. Moreover, retinoids also seem to block the activity of activator protein-1 (AP-1), whose potential role in the induction of matrix metalloproteinases (MMPs) and the pathogenesis of acne and acne scarring was discussed in the previous chapter (Darwiche *et al.* 2005; Huang *et al.* 1997; Uchida *et al.* 2003).

Additionally, tretinoin, but not the other synthetic retinoids, has been found to bind cytosolic retinoic acid-binding proteins I and II (CRABP-I and -II). The function of these proteins was previously thought to only include the transport and buffering of retinoic acid in the cell (Dong *et al.* 1999); however, they may also be directly involved in the cellular proliferation and differentiation pathways (Shroot 1998). Most recently, tretinoin and adapalene have been found to down-regulate the expression of Toll-like receptor (TLR)-2 *in vitro* (Liu *et al.* 2005; Tenaud *et al.* 2007). As discussed in the previous chapter, TLR-2 may be a key activator of the immune response in acne. These *in vitro* findings will need to be confirmed in clinical studies.

Although numerous adverse effects may result from the use of oral retinoids (as will be demonstrated in the case of oral isotretinoin below), topical retinoids are mostly associated with application-site reactions (14). Systemic absorption of topically-applied retinoids is low and varies from 0.01% for adapalene to 1–2% for tretinoin and to less than 1% for tazarotene when applied without occlusion or 6% when applied with occlusion (Allec *et al.* 1997; Latriano *et al.* 1997; Menter 2000; Tang-Liu *et al.* 1999; Yu *et al.* 2003). Localized pruritus, burning, erythema, and scaling may occur with all topical retinoids, but appear to be least pronounced with adapalene and stronger with tazarotene, possibly reflecting their relative depth of penetration into the epidermis (Cunliffe *et al.* 1998; Leyden *et al.* 2001c). Although not available worldwide, the microsphere delivery of tretinoin and the incorporation of tretinoin molecules into a polyolprepolymer-2 gel seem to result in greater retention of the active ingredient within the stratum corneum and subsequent decreased rates of local irritation (Berger *et al.* 2007; Skov *et al.* 1997). Of note, application-site reactions tend to improve with continued use. Patients should also be warned about the risk of the so-called 'retinoid flare', an exacerbation in acne severity, which may occur in the first weeks of treatment with gradual resolution thereafter.

Topical retinoids have not been shown to interact with any oral agents; however, greater application-site irritation may occur with topical regimens that include benzoyl peroxide and salicylic acid. Also, as mentioned in a previous section, the conventional formulations of topical tretinoin, but not the microsphere formulation or the newer retinoids adapalene and tazarotene, are rapidly inactivated in the presence of benzoyl peroxide (Martin *et al.* 1998; Nyirady *et al.* 2002; Shroot 1998).

Topical tretinoin and adapalene are both FDA pregnancy category C agents, whereas topical tazarotene has been designated as pregnancy category X. Thus, the use of topical tazarotene is prohibited during pregnancy and proper contraception has to be utilized at all times. It may be noted, however, that reports of pregnancies occurring during treatment with topical tazarotene did not document any congenital abnormalities (Weinstein *et al.* 1997). The excretion of topically-applied retinoids in human breast milk has not been adequately studied, and their use during lactation is not recommended.

Azelaic acid

Azelaic acid is a naturally-occurring 9-carbon-chain dicarboxylic acid derived from *Pityrosporum ovale*, but also found in cereals and animal products. It is commercially available as a 20% cream and a 15% gel, with the latter formulation currently FDA-approved only for rosacea. In the treatment of acne vulgaris, azelaic acid is typically applied twice daily.

When utilized in the treatment of acne, azelaic acid appears to have antiproliferative and antikeratinizing properties (Mayer-da-Silva *et al.* 1989). In addition, its

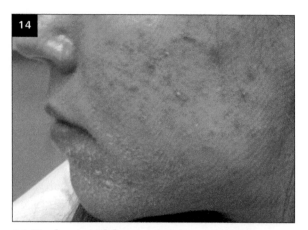

14 Erythema and desquamation are commonly encountered with excessive use of a topical retinoid.

antibacterial effect has also been demonstrated and may at least in part be due to the perturbation of the intracellular pH and subsequent inhibition of protein synthesis (Bladon *et al.* 1986; Bojar *et al.* 1991; Bojar *et al.* 1994). In addition, azelaic acid is a reversible inhibitor of tyrosinase, a rate-limiting enzyme central to melanin synthesis. This effect is selective, as highly active melanocytes are preferentially affected by the compound (Robins *et al.* 1985). Consequently, azelaic acid is sometimes also used in the treatment of acne vulgaris associated with hyperpigmentation (**15**).

Systemic absorption following a single topical application of the 20% cream formulation is less than 4%, but increases to 8% when the 15% gel is used (Fitton & Goa 1991; Tauber *et al.* 1992). This results in negligible variations in the normal baseline serum levels as determined by dietary consumption. Consequently, only localized application-site adverse effects have been reported with azelaic acid. These most commonly include pruritus, burning, erythema, and peeling. Topical azelaic acid has not been reported to interact with any oral medications. Azelaic acid is an FDA pregnancy category B agent. Since azelaic acid from dietary intake is excreted in breast milk, it is unlikely that topically-applied agent would significantly alter its level during lactation.

Sulfur

Sulfur is a nonmetallic chemical element long used in the treatment of acne vulgaris, among other conditions. It is available in numerous formulations and concentrations ranging from 1% to 10% and is frequently combined with sodium sulfacetamide, benzoyl peroxide, resorcinol, or salicylic acid for a synergistic effect. In the treatment of acne vulgaris, such preparations are typically used once to three times daily. However, in the UK sulfur preparations are not commercially available.

Sulfur is thought to interact with cysteine in the stratum corneum to form hydrogen sulfide, although the exact mechanism of such interaction has not been completely elucidated. Hydrogen sulfide breaks down keratin, leading to the keratolytic effect of topically-applied sulfur. In addition, sulfur appears to have an inhibitory effect on the growth of *P. acnes* bacteria, possibly from the inactivation of sulfhydryl groups in the bacterial enzymes (Gupta & Nicol 2004).

Systemic absorption following topical application has been estimated to be around 1% (Lin *et al.* 1988). Topical administration may result in localized adverse effects, including mild erythema and peeling. Aside from these adverse effects, the malodor associated with sulfur is frequently a limiting factor in the use of this agent in patients. It has not been reported to interact with any systemic agents. Of note, elemental sulfur does not cross-react with sulfonamides and can thus be used in sulfonamide-sensitive patients. Sulfur is an FDA pregnancy category C agent and its excretion in breast milk has not been studied.

Sodium sulfacetamide

Sodium sulfacetamide is a sulfonamide antibacterial agent used in some countries alone or in combination with sulfur. Most preparations utilize 10% sodium sulfacetamide and 5% sulfur and are available as suspensions, lotions, or creams, as well as in the form of cleansers. Like other sulfonamides, sodium sulfacetamide is a competitive antagonist to para-aminobenzoic acid (PABA), which is essential for bacterial growth (Gupta & Nicol 2004).

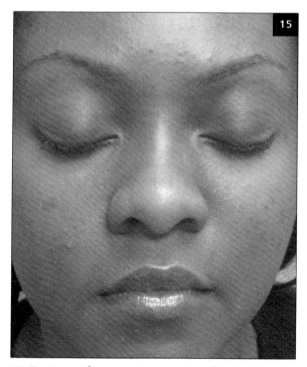

15 Patient with concomitant acne and postinflammatory hyperpigmentation would be a good candidate for topical azelaic acid therapy.

Adverse effects from topically-applied sodium sulfacetamide typically include local pruritus and erythema. Although not reported with cutaneous use, topical sulfacetamide has, on occasion, led to the development of erythema multiforme or even Stevens–Johnson syndrome when applied via the ophthalmic route (Genvert et al. 1985; Gottschalk & Stone 1976; Rubin 1977). It is contraindicated in patients with a history of sensitivity to sulfonamides, commonly referred to as 'sulfa drugs'. Although orally-administered sulfonamides may result in various, occasionally life-threatening, adverse effects and numerous drug interactions, these have not been reported with topical sodium sulfacetamide use.

Sodium sulfacetamide is an FDA pregnancy category C agent. Its excretion in breast milk has not been studied. However, because of the risk of kernicterus in nursing infants with the use of systemic sulfonamides (Wennberg & Ahlfors 2006), topical use during lactation is not advised.

ORAL AGENTS

Common indications for the initiation of oral therapy for acne vulgaris include patients with moderate to severe acne, patients with acne resistant to topical therapy, patients with acne prone to scarring, and patients with truncal involvement.

Antibiotics

Tetracyclines are some of the most commonly used oral antibiotics in the treatment of acne vulgaris. These include tetracycline (oxytetracycline and tetracycline hydrochloride), doxycycline, and minocycline. Lymecycline, a second-generation tetracycline with improved oral absorption and slower elimination than tetracycline, is used outside the US and will not be discussed further in this chapter (Dubertret et al. 2003).

Tetracycline is available as 250 mg or 500 mg tablets or capsules, and is most commonly initiated at 500 mg twice daily, followed by 500 mg daily once the condition improves. Doxycycline is available in numerous formulations, including capsules, tablets, and enteric-coated tablets, with dosages ranging from 20 mg twice daily (subantimicrobial dose) to 100 mg twice daily. In addition, capsules containing 30 mg of immediate-release and 10 mg of delayed-release doxycycline have been FDA-approved for rosacea, but are sometimes used off-label for the treatment of acne

vulgaris. Minocycline is available as capsules and tablets, with doses ranging from 50 to 100 mg twice daily. An extended-release minocycline tablet has been approved by the FDA for the treatment of moderate to severe acne vulgaris and is typically administered in doses of 1 mg/kg (Stewart et al. 2006).

All three agents have a tetracyclic naphthacene carboxamide ring structure and bind divalent and polyvalent metal cations, such as calcium and magnesium (Sapadin & Fleischmajer 2006). As antibiotic agents, tetracyclines are bacteriostatic and act by binding to the 30S ribosomal subunit, thereby inhibiting protein synthesis. It is thought that this results in the inhibition of bacterial lipases, with subsequent reduction in the antigenic free fatty acid content of the sebum. Additionally, tetracyclines have been found to have important anti-inflammatory effects, whose contribution to the improvement of acne vulgaris may potentially be even greater than that of their antibiotic properties. As such, tetracyclines have been demonstrated to suppress neutrophil chemotaxis, to inhibit collagenases and gelatinase, also known as MMPs, to inhibit the formation of reactive oxygen species, to up-regulate anti-inflammatory cytokines, and to down-regulate proinflammatory cytokines (Amin et al. 1996; Esterly et al. 1978, 1984; Golub et al. 1995; Kloppenburg et al. 1995; Lee et al. 1982; Sainte-Marie et al. 1999; Yao et al. 2004, 2007). Minocycline and doxycycline have also been shown to have antiangiogenic properties, possibly through the inhibition of MMP synthesis by endothelial cells, although this effect is likely more relevant to the treatment of rosacea than of acne vulgaris (Guerin et al. 1992; Tamargo et al. 1991; Yao et al. 2007). The anti-inflammatory properties of tetracyclines have been compared with the subantimicrobial dosing of doxycycline, found to be effective in the treatment of acne while avoiding microbial resistance and alteration of cutaneous flora (Skidmore et al. 2003).

The absorption of tetracycline is decreased by about 50% when taken with food; thus, it should be taken 1 hour before or 2 hours after a meal. On the other hand, doxycycline and minocycline absorption is unaffected by food. In addition, because of their ability to bind divalent metals, the absorption of tetracyclines from the gastrointestinal tract is lowered with concurrent ingestion of dairy products, antacids containing calcium, aluminum, or magnesium, and iron and zinc salts (Healy et al. 1997; Neuvonen 1976). The serum half-life of tetracycline is 8.5 hours, whereas doxycycline and minocycline are longer-lasting, with half-lives of 12–25 hours and 12–18 hours, respectively (Agwuh & MacGowan 2006; Sadick 2007). Tetracycline is excreted renally (Phillips *et al.* 1974), whereas doxycycline and, to a slightly lesser extent, minocycline are excreted primarily through the gastrointestinal tract and are, therefore, generally safe for use in renal failure (Agwuh & MacGowan 2006).

The most common adverse effects associated with tetracyclines are gastrointestinal and may include heartburn, nausea, vomiting, diarrhea, and, less commonly, esophagitis and esophageal ulcerations. Photosensitivity is most common with doxycycline and may be associated with photo-onycholysis. On the other hand, central nervous system complaints, most commonly vertigo, are often noted with the use of minocycline. Vaginal candidiasis is another common adverse effect of tetracyclines. Hypersensitivity reactions, ranging from exanthems to urticaria with pneumonitis to Stevens–Johnson syndrome have all been described, but are more frequent with minocycline (Smith & Leyden 2005). In children, the deposition of tetracyclines in teeth and bones may result in tooth discoloration and delayed growth; thus, the use of tetracyclines in children under 8 years of age and in pregnant women should be avoided. In addition, minocycline may cause bluish discoloration of scars and areas of prior inflammation, bluish-gray pigmentation of normal skin of the shins and forearms, muddy brown discoloration in sun-exposed locations, as well as bluish-gray discoloration of the sclerae, oral mucosa, tongue, teeth, and nails and black discoloration of the thyroid gland (Angeloni *et al.* 1987; Mouton *et al.* 2004, Oertel 2007).

Less common, but serious, adverse effects associated with the use of oral tetracyclines include nephrotoxicity, hepatotoxicity and autoimmune hepatitis, hemolytic anemia, thrombocytopenia, serum sickness-like syndrome, and increased intracranial pressure (pseudotumor cerebri), especially if administered simultaneously with oral retinoids or vitamin A (Bihorac *et al.* 1999; D'Addario *et al.* 2003; Friedman 2005; Lawrenson *et al.* 2000; Lewis & Kearney 1997; Shapiro *et al.* 1997). Minocycline has also been implicated in drug-induced lupus erythematosus and polyarteritis nodosa (Margolis *et al.* 2007; Pelletier *et al.* 2003; Schaffer *et al.* 2001; Shapiro *et al.* 1997).

Several drug interactions have been described with tetracyclines. As previously mentioned, antacids, laxatives, oral supplements, and dairy products containing divalent and polyvalent metals reduce the absorption of tetracyclines and their concurrent use should be avoided. In addition, antacids, including H_2 blockers and proton pump inhibitors, increase pH in the stomach and may decrease gastrointestinal absorption of tetracyclines. Tetracyclines may increase the serum levels of digoxin, lithium, and warfarin; thus, the levels of these agents should be carefully monitored to prevent toxicity. Tetracyclines may reduce insulin requirements and have been reported to cause hypoglycemia. Finally, anticonvulsants, including phenytoin, barbiturates, and carbamazepine, may reduce the half-life of doxycycline, but not the other tetracyclines (Sadick 2007). Because of the previously-mentioned adverse effects on the developing teeth and bones, tetracyclines are designated as FDA pregnancy category D. As well, these agents are excreted in breast milk and should not be used in nursing mothers.

Azithromycin, a methyl derivative of erythromycin, is a macrolide antibiotic, which inhibits protein synthesis by binding to the 50S bacterial ribosomal subunit. It is available as 250 mg, 500 mg, and 600 mg tablets, 250 mg and 500 mg capsules, as powder for oral suspension, and as an extended-release oral suspension. Although currently not FDA-approved for the treatment of acne vulgaris, azithromycin has been investigated for off-label use in this condition and found to be at least as efficacious as tetracyclines (Kus *et al.* 2005; Parsad *et al.* 2001; Rafiei & Yaghoobi 2006). The pharmacokinetic profile of azithromycin is characterized by a rapid uptake into tissues from serum and a long tissue half-life of 60–72 hours (Crokaert *et al.* 1998; Neu 1991). Numerous regimens have been proposed and additional studies will need to determine the optimal dosing schedule of this emerging therapeutic option.

The most common adverse effects associated with azithromycin include nausea and diarrhea, although their incidence is significantly lower compared to that encountered with oral erythromycin, as is the incidence of candidal vaginitis (Fernandez-Obregon 2000). Azithromycin is an FDA pregnancy category B agent. The safety of azithromycin in pregnancy constitutes a potential advantage over tetracyclines in the corresponding population.

Trimethoprim with or without sulfamethoxazole is a third-line agent used off-label in the treatment of acne vulgaris resistant to other oral antibiotics (Cunliffe et al. 1999) (16, 17). Singly, trimethoprim is available as 100 mg and 200 mg tablets. The combined trimethoprim–sulfamethoxazole, also known as co-trimoxazole, is available as a single-strength tablet, containing 80 mg of trimethoprim and 400 mg of sulfamethoxazole, or a double-strength tablet, with double the amount of each of the component agents. Several dosing regimens exist, with trimethoprim typically administered as 100 mg three times daily or 300 mg twice daily, and co-trimoxazole typically administered as two single-strength tablets or one double-strength tablet twice daily.

The action of sulfamethoxazole and trimethoprim is synergistic, as the agents block consecutive steps in the bacterial synthesis of folic acid and tetrahydrofolate, necessary for the synthesis of nucleic acids. It has also been proposed that the follicular concentration of trimethoprim, unlike other commonly used oral antibiotics, is unaffected by elevated sebum excretion rates (Layton et al. 1992). This may explain, in part, the therapeutic success occasionally observed with this agent despite previous failures with other oral antibiotics. Once absorbed, the half-lives of trimethoprim and sulfamethoxazole are 11 and 9 hours, respectively, but may be increased in renal failure (Sadick 2007).

The use of co-trimoxazole in the treatment of acne has been limited by the perceived high incidence of severe adverse effects, most notably toxic epidermal necrolysis. An extensive review of patient data indicates, however, that the incidence of this and other serious adverse effects, such as Stevens–Johnson syndrome, severe blood count abnormalities, and renal or hepatic dysfunction, is likely to be low (Jick & Derby 1995). Since sulfamethoxazole is a sulfonamide, co-trimoxazole, but not trimethoprim alone, is contraindicated in patients with documented history of allergies to 'sulfa' medications. As with other sulfonamides, sulfamethoxazole may cause kernicterus in newborns (Wennberg & Ahlfors 2006).

Most common adverse effects include a morbilliform or fixed-drug eruption and urticaria. Additional common adverse effects include gastrointestinal complaints, such as nausea and vomiting, dizziness, headaches, and candidal vaginitis (Cunliffe et al. 1999). Co-trimoxazole can rarely induce hemolytic anemia in patients with glucose-6-phosphate dehydrogenase (G6PD) deficiency and trigger an attack of porphyria in predisposed patients (Chan 1997). Although uncommon, trimethoprim and co-trimoxazole can lead to folate deficiency with subsequent megaloblastic anemia and granulocytopenia (Cunliffe et al. 1999).

Co-trimoxazole may displace serum albumin-bound warfarin and thus potentiate its anticoagulant effect (Campbell & Carter 2005). Concurrent administration of methotrexate and co-trimoxazole should be avoided due to an increased risk of myelosuppression (Groenendal & Rampen 1990; Thomas et al. 1987). In addition, digoxin and phenytoin levels may become elevated when co-administered with co-trimoxazole and should be carefully monitored.

Both trimethoprim and sulfamethoxazole are FDA pregnancy category C agents, as they may interfere with folic acid metabolism; in addition, sulfamethoxazole may cause kernicterus in the fetus when administered during the third trimester. Both agents are expressed in breast milk and should not be used during lactation due to the risk of adverse effects in the infant.

Isotretinoin

Isotretinoin, or 13-cis retinoic acid, is a first-generation retinoid that has been available in Europe since 1971 and FDA-approved for the treatment of severe nodulocystic acne since 1982. In the treatment of acne and related conditions, isotretinoin is also used in patients with recalcitrant acne (18, 19), those who are prone to severe acne scarring, and in patients with Gram-negative folliculitis. Isotretinoin is available as 5 mg, 10 mg, 20 mg, 30 mg, and 40 mg capsules, and is typically administered daily with meals that include fatty foods to enhance gastrointestinal absorption. Various dosing regimens have been attempted over the years, with the most common one being 0.5–1.0 mg/kg/day for 6–12 months to reach a total cumulative dose of 120–150 mg/kg. Higher doses, up to 2.0 mg/kg/day, may be required for recalcitrant cases or severe truncal acne. Additional newer developments have included low-dose long-term isotretinoin administration, with dosages as low as 10–20 mg daily, and various intermittent regimens (Akman et al. 2007; Amichai et al. 2006; Goulden et al. 1997; Kaymak & Ilter 2006). Such regimens, however, are associated with a higher risk of relapse following the discontinuation of the medication.

Isotretinoin is the most potent inhibitor of sebum production. The mechanism of this action is not entirely clear. In fact, isotretinoin has not demonstrated clear

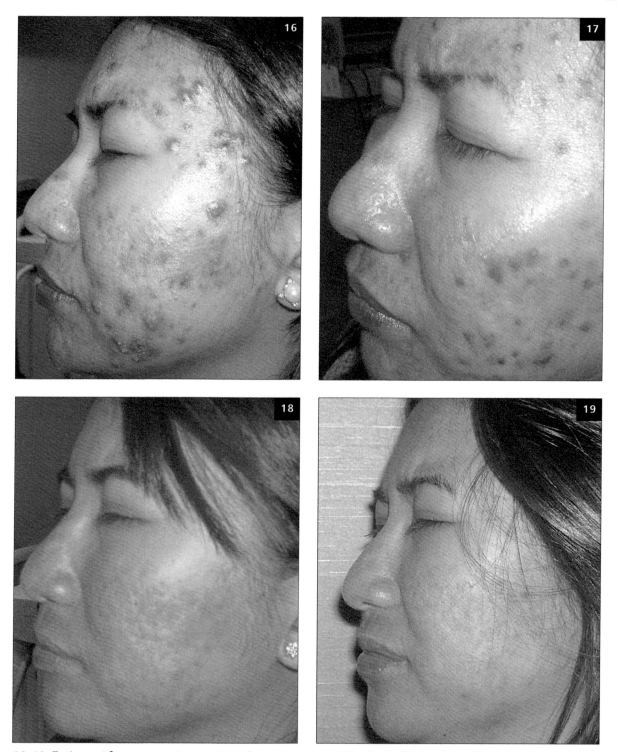

16–19 **Patient with severe cystic acne. 16** Before treatment. **17** After 1 month of oral trimethoprim–sulfamethoxazole, showing only mild improvement. **18** After 3 months of oral isotretinoin. **19** At the completion of a 6-month regimen of oral isotretinoin, showing excellent response.

affinity for any of the RAR or RXR subtypes (see the above discussion of topical retinoids). It has been suggested that intracellular isomerization to all-*trans* retinoic acid may be involved in sebosuppression (Tsukada *et al*. 2000). Alternatively, the effect of isotretinoin on sebocytes may be independent of the retinoid receptors. Isotretinoin has been shown to reduce androgen receptor-binding capacity and the formation of dihydrotestosterone, which regulates sebum production (Boudou *et al*. 1994, 1995). RAR-independent cell-cycle arrest and apoptosis have been demonstrated in sebocytes exposed to isotretinoin (Nelson *et al*. 2006).

Once absorbed, isotretinoin is mostly bound to albumin in plasma. Its elimination half-life is approximately 20 hours and, unlike vitamin A and fat-soluble retinoids, isotretinoin is not stored in the liver or the adipose tissue. The metabolism of isotretinoin occurs mainly in the liver, where it is oxidized to 4-oxo-isotretinoin. In addition, tretinoin and its metabolite, 4-oxo-tretinoin, may also be produced in smaller amounts. Isotretinoin and its metabolites are then excreted in urine and feces, reaching their naturally-occurring concentrations within 2 weeks following the discontinuation of the agent (Allen & Bloxham 1989).

Numerous adverse effects are associated with the use of oral isotretinoin. Many of the side-effects resemble clinical manifestations of hypervitaminosis A. The most serious adverse effect is retinoid teratogenicity, which recently prompted the launch of a mandatory online compliance program in the US. Fetal exposure to isotretinoin may cause stillbirths or spontaneous abortions. Nearly 50% of the infants exposed to the agent during the first trimester and delivered at full term are affected, with the most common abnormalities being auditory (microtia, conductive or sensorineural hearing loss), cardiovascular (septal defects, overriding aorta, tetralogy of Fallot, hypoplastic aortic arch), craniofacial and musculoskeletal (cleft palate, jaw malformation, micrognathia, bony aplasia and hypoplasia), ocular (microphthalmia, atrophy of the optic nerve), central neural (cortical agenesis, hydrocephalus, microcephaly), and thymic (aplasia or hypoplasia) (Lammer *et al*. 1985; Stern *et al*. 1984). Since there is no established teratogenic threshold for isotretinoin, females of child-bearing potential have to be counseled on pregnancy prevention, with two forms of contraception being mandatory for the initiation of therapy. As well, the proper use of contraception must be ascertained at each monthly visit. Two negative serum or urine pregnancy tests are mandatory in the US prior to starting oral isotretinoin. In addition, a pregnancy test has to be repeated monthly for the duration of therapy, as well as 1 month following the discontinuation of treatment to allow for the washout period.

Common mucocutaneous adverse effects of oral isotretinoin include dryness of the lips, mouth, nose, and eyes. Mucosal dryness and fragility can then lead to epistaxis, conjunctivitis, corneal ulcerations, and superinfections with *Staphylococcus aureus* (Aragona *et al*. 2005; Azurdia & Sharpe 1999; Bozkurt *et al*. 2002; Shalita 1987). Additional ophthalmologic findings may include altered night vision and photophobia (Halpagi *et al*. 2008).

Xerosis of the skin and photosensitivity are frequently observed, as are nail fragility and occasional telogen effluvium. In addition, an elevated incidence of delayed wound healing and keloidal scar formation following surgical or laser procedures on patients taking oral isotretinoin has been noted (Bernstein & Geronemus 1997; Zachariae 1988). This may be related to the previously mentioned modulation of MMP expression by retinoids; specifically, lower expression of collagenases may lead to excessive scar tissue deposition (Abergel *et al*. 1985). Excessive granulation tissue with subsequent keloid formation has also been observed in severe cases of acne conglobata and acne fulminans upon initiation of isotretinoin therapy. For this reason, pretreatment with systemic corticosteroids for up to 6 weeks is recommended in such instances (Seukeran & Cunliffe 1999). Additionally, acne flares varying in severity from mild to severe, including acne fulminans, have been reported with oral isotretinoin (Chivot 2001, Lehucher Ceyrac et al. 1998).

The most common musculoskeletal adverse effects include bone pain, as well as myalgia and muscle cramps, especially after strenuous exercise. Most of these complaints are minor and have no long-term sequelae. Several reports suggest, but do not definitively prove, an association between long-term use of isotretinoin and the development of diffuse idiopathic skeletal hyperostosis (DISH) syndrome, characterized by the formation of largely asymptomatic hyperostoses of the spine, as well as calcification of tendons and ligaments, such as that of the anterior spinal ligament (DiGiovanna 2001; Ling et al. 2001). Children on high-dose, long-term oral isotretinoin can develop premature partial epiphyseal closure (Nishimura et al. 1997). On the other hand, isotretinoin does not appear to induce osteoporosis or other abnormalities of bone mineral density (DiGiovanna et al. 2004).

Adverse effects involving the central nervous system are exceedingly rare. However, a complaint of persistent headache, especially when accompanied by nausea, vomiting, and blurry vision, should prompt an immediate ophthalmologic evaluation to rule out papilledema associated with pseudotumor cerebri (Roytman et al. 1988). This complication is most common when isotretinoin is co-administered with oral tetracyclines; thus, their concurrent use should be avoided (Lee 1995).

The association between oral isotretinoin intake and psychiatric disturbances, most notably depression and suicidal ideation, has been highly controversial. Although several reports have appeared in the literature (Scheinman et al. 1990), it has been argued that some patients with severe and debilitating acne requiring oral isotretinoin may have baseline depressive symptoms prior to therapy. As of now, extensive reviews fail to establish a causative association (Chia et al. 2005; Hull & D'Arcy 2005; Jick et al. 2000; Marqueling & Zane 2007).

Serious gastrointestinal and hepatic adverse effects are rare, although nausea, diarrhea, and mild transient elevation of transaminases are somewhat more common. Liver function tests should be obtained at baseline; however, it is unclear whether additional tests at follow-up visits are necessary (Alcalay et al. 2001; Barth et al. 1993). If laboratory monitoring of liver function is undertaken, the medication should be temporarily withheld if two- to threefold elevation in hepatic enzymes is noted, and discontinued if greater than threefold elevation is documented. On rare occasion, a flare of inflammatory bowel syndrome in patients treated with oral isotretinoin has been reported; however, the causal relationship has not been demonstrated in prospective studies (Godfrey & James

1990; Reddy et al. 2006). Finally, several cases of pancreatitis associated with isotretinoin-induced hyperlipidemia have been reported, suggesting the need for further investigations in patients with abdominal pain while on the medication (Flynn et al. 1987; McCarter & Chen 1992).

Lipid profile abnormalities, primarily hyper-triglyceridemia and hypercholesterolemia, are common during oral isotretinoin therapy (Zane et al. 2006). Most cases do not require clinical intervention; however, dietary adjustments and the addition of lipid-lowering agents, such as gemfibrozil, may be considered in some patients. It is recommended that lipid profile be monitored monthly for 3–6 months and every 3 months thereafter. Triglyceride or cholesterol elevation above 6.78 mmol/l (600 mg/dl) or 7.7 mmol/l (300 mg/dl), respectively, should prompt a temporary withholding of the medication until the values are normalized.

Blood count abnormalities are rare; however, leukopenia and occasional agranulocytosis have been reported with the use of oral isotretinoin (Friedman 1987; Ozdemir et al. 2007; Waisman 1988). Because of the relative paucity of such adverse effects, the optimal hematologic monitoring schedule, if any, is not clear, except in patients with human immunodeficiency virus (HIV), in whom frequent testing is recommended.

Toxicity from oral isotretinoin may be increased by concurrent administration of vitamin A supplementation. As previously mentioned, the risk of pseudotumor cerebri is significantly elevated when tetracyclines and isotretinoin are combined. Additionally, various inhibitors of CYP 3A4, a hepatic enzyme involved in the metabolism of isotretinoin, are expected to elevate the serum level of the agent. On the other hand, inducers of the enzyme, including rifamin and anticonvulsants, may decrease isotretinoin to subtherapeutic levels. Concurrent administration with methotrexate is not recommended due to the combined risk of hepatotoxicity.

Because of its severe teratogenic potential, oral isotretinoin is an FDA pregnancy category X agent, and its use in the US is tightly regulated through the previously-mentioned online monitoring system. Isotretinoin is absolutely contraindicated in nursing mothers.

Hormonal therapies

Hormonal agents may be used in women for the treatment of acne regardless of the baseline serum androgen levels. They are especially useful in inflammatory acne resistant to oral antibiotics and in women with significant flares prior to their menstrual periods. Hormonal therapies used in the treatment of acne in women are divided into inhibitors of androgen production and androgen receptor blockers.

The most commonly used inhibitors of androgen production are oral contraceptives. Agents used in the treatment of acne are comprised of a combination of an estrogen, typically ethinyl estradiol, and a synthetic progestin. Of the progestins, the first-generation agents, such as norgestrel, have an intrinsically high affinity for androgen receptors. The second-generation agents are associated with lower androgenicity and include norethindrone, levonorgestrel, and ethynodiol diacetate. The newest synthetic progestins have very low or no androgenic potential and include desogestrel, norgestimate, gestodene (currently only available outside the US), and drospirenone (a spironolactone analog with antiandrogenic and antimineralocorticoid activity). Additionally, an oral contraceptive agent consisting of ethinyl estradiol and cyproterone acetate, a derivative of 17-hydroxyprogesterone with antiandrogenic properties and weak progestational activity, is currently available outside the US. Both the combined contraceptive and singular formulations of cyproterone acetate have been successfully used in the treatment of acne (Beylot et al. 1998).

At higher doses, estrogen can suppress sebum production. However, because of a higher incidence of adverse effects associated with such doses, the current trend has been to lower estrogen content to 20–35 μg per dose. At these levels, the mechanism of action appears to be increased liver production of sex hormone-binding globulin, with subsequent decrease in the circulating levels of free testosterone, and decreased adrenal and ovarian androgen production through negative feedback and suppression of ovulation (Coenen et al. 1996; Wiegratz et al. 1995).

The most common adverse effects associated with the use of oral contraceptive agents include nausea, headaches, weight gain, abnormal menses, mood changes, and breast tenderness. Extensive epidemiological studies have investigated the risk of the more serious adverse effects of oral contraceptives, including venous thromboembolic events, myocardial infarction, and stroke. These studies confirmed that the risk of myocardial infarction and stroke is not elevated in the users of oral contraceptives containing less than 50 μg of ethinyl estradiol. The exception to this finding is smokers over the age of 35 years, in whom the risk is unacceptably high and who should not, therefore, be prescribed combined oral contraceptives. All oral contraceptives have been found to carry a small, but measurable, excess risk of venous thromboembolism. In addition, it appears that the use of agents containing desogestrel or gestodene doubles this risk; however, no cause-and-effect association has been established (Carr & Ory 1997; Jick et al. 1995, 2006; Lewis et al. 1997). Although some analyses seem to indicate an association between long-term use of oral contraceptives and slightly elevated risk of breast, cervical, and hepatocellular cancers, these findings remain controversial (Cogliano et al. 2005; Shapiro & Szarewski 2007; Szarewski 2005).

Failure of oral contraceptives in the prevention of pregnancy may occur when co-administered with inducers of hepatic cytochrome P-450 enzyme, such as phenobarbital, rifampin, and griseofulvin. Although isolated reports suggested a possible reduction in contraceptive efficacy in the presence of oral antibiotics such as tetracyclines, the actual failure rate is no greater than the one expected in the general population (Dickinson et al. 2001; Helms et al. 1997).

Spironolactone is a synthetic steroid most resembling mineralocorticoids. It is FDA-approved for diuresis for various indications. It has, however, also been used off-label for the treatment of acne for over 20 years (Burke & Cunliffe 1985; Goodfellow et al. 1984; Shaw 2000). It is available as 25 mg, 50 mg, and 100 mg tablets. Additionally, topical cream and lotion preparations containing 5% spironolactone are available in some countries outside of the U.S. and the U.K.. Dosages most commonly utilized in the treatment of acne are 50–200 mg per day, which may be subdivided into morning and evening doses for lower incidence of adverse effects.

Spironolactone is primarily an aldosterone antagonist that is also a progestin, a weak androgen receptor blocker, and an inhibitor of androgen synthesis. In addition, spironolactone inhibits the enzyme 5α-reductase, responsible for the conversion of testosterone to dihydrotestosterone, and significantly reduces sebum production (Goodfellow et al. 1984). While the oral bioavailability of the agent is good, its gastrointestinal absorption may be further improved by co-administration with food (Overdiek & Merkus 1986). Spironolactone is metabolized in the liver to several active metabolites, including 7α-thiomethylspironolactone, canrenone, and 6β-hydroxy-7α- thiomethylspironolactone, which are then excreted in urine and bile (Overdiek et al. 1985).

Although adverse effects are common with spironolactone, occurring in up to 90% of patients, most are mild and without long-term sequelae (Shaw 2000; Shaw & White 2002; Yemisci et al. 2005). While diuresis is an expected occurrence with the use of oral spironolactone in the treatment of acne, common adverse effects include fatigue, headaches, vertigo, menstrual irregularities, and breast tenderness. Most incidences of menstrual irregularities frequently resolve spontaneously over 2–3 months; however, an oral contraceptive may be added if the symptoms are bothersome to the patient (Burke & Cunliffe 1985). Most adverse effects are dose-dependent and may improve or resolve completely with lower dosages (Shaw 2000).

Less common adverse effects include nausea, vomiting, confusion, decreased libido, orthostatic hypotension, and hyperkalemia. Clinically-significant hyperkalemia is unlikely in young healthy women, but may be of potential concern in older patients, those with renal insufficiency, or with concurrent administration of oral potassium supplementation. Specific monitoring guidelines for serum potassium are lacking because of the low risk of this complication; if considered, potassium level may be checked at baseline and repeated early into therapy. It is also important to note that the FDA has placed a warning on the package insert of spironolactone, as neoplastic potential in rats has been demonstrated with extremely high doses of the agent. Although a concern about breast cancer risk in patients on oral spironolactone has been raised on one occasion, the risk has subsequently been shown to be equivalent to the one in the general population (Danielson et al. 1982; Friedman & Ury 1980; Loube & Quirk 1975; Shaw & White 2002).

Although relatively few drug interactions are clinically important, the risk of hyperkalemia from the use of oral spironolactone is increased when the agent is administered concurrently with potassium supplements or angiotensin-converting enzyme inhibitors. Serum concentration of digoxin and lithium may increase to potentially toxic levels when co-administered with spironolactone and should, therefore, be carefully monitored. Spironolactone is an FDA pregnancy category C agent and should not be administered during pregnancy due to the risk of feminization of a male fetus. Oral contraceptives represent a convenient approach to decrease the risk of pregnancy and to add to the clinical efficacy of spironolactone in clearing acne. The active metabolites of spironolactone have been detected in breast milk; thus, its use in nursing mothers is discouraged (Phelps & Karim 1977).

Additional hormonal therapies occasionally tried in the treatment of acne vulgaris include flutamide, a nonsteroidal antagonist of the androgen receptor, leuprolide and other gonadotropin-releasing hormone agonists, and finasteride, an inhibitor of 5α-reductase type II. At the present time, solid data from large clinical trials supporting such use are lacking for these agents; future studies may confirm or refute their clinical benefit in this condition.

3 LASERS AND SIMILAR DEVICES IN THE TREATMENT OF ACNE VULGARIS

INTRODUCTION

IN addition to the numerous medical therapeutic options available for acne vulgaris introduced in the previous chapter, multiple lasers and laser-like devices have been found to be of substantial clinical value in the treatment of this common condition. The devices and techniques described in this chapter now have a considerable track record of clinical efficacy and safety, and may be used alone or, for the best results, concurrently with medical therapeutic agents.

MID-INFRARED RANGE LASERS

Originally developed for nonablative photorejuvenation of the skin, several mid-infrared lasers have subsequently been found to be of significant use in the treatment of acne vulgaris (**20, 21**) and, as will be discussed in the next chapter, acne scarring. These include the 1320-nm neodymium:yttrium-aluminum-garnet (Nd:YAG) laser (CoolTouch CT3, CoolTouch Corp,

Roseville, CA, USA), the 1450-nm diode laser (SmoothBeam, Candela Corp, Wayland, MA, USA), and the 1540-nm ytterbium-erbium:phosphate glass, also known as erbium:glass (Er:glass) laser (Aramis, Quantel Derma GmbH, Erlangen, Germany) (*Table 2*).

Name	Manufacturer	Wavelength (nm)	Cooling
CoolTouch CT3	CoolTouch	1320	Cryogen
ThermaScan	Sciton	1319	Contact
SmoothBeam	Candela	1450	Cryogen
Aramis	Quantel Derma	1540	Contact

Table 2 Examples of commercially-available mid-infrared lasers

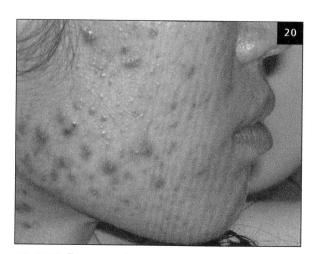
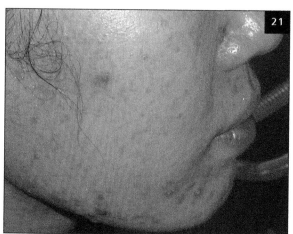

20, 21 **Inflammatory acne in an Asian patient. 20** Before treatment. **21** Following two sessions with a 1320-nm laser.

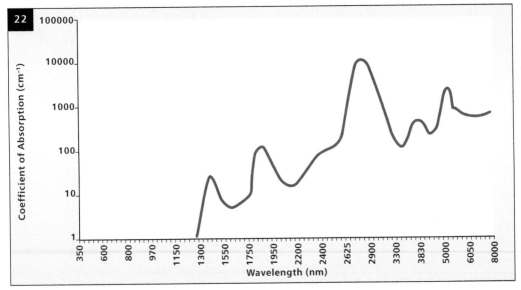

22 Light absorption spectrum of water.

Mechanism of action

Although the exact details of the mechanism of action of mid-infrared lasers in the treatment of acne vulgaris have not been elucidated, ongoing research is being performed. All three wavelengths are well absorbed by water, resulting in bulk heating of the dermis as heat is propagated from the dermal water content (**22**). The laser beam emitted by each of the three systems is known to penetrate to the level of the sebaceous glands in the skin, typically located at 200–1000 μm below the stratum corneum (Dahan *et al.* 2004; Paithankar *et al.* 2002). Of note, light at 1320 nm is least absorbed by water and, consequently, has the greatest optical penetration depth in the skin, defined as the depth at which laser energy is attenuated through absorption and scattering to 1/e, or approximately 37%, of the original value.

From the study of the 1450-nm wavelength, it appears that at least one mechanism of action of the mid-infrared lasers may be functional, if not structural, alteration of the sebaceous glands. In the study by Paithankar *et al.* (2002), thermal coagulation of the sebaceous lobule was demonstrated in rabbit and human skin immediately following laser irradiation. Biopsies obtained from h uman subjects at 2 and 6 months following treatment, however, showed normal sebaceous glands and ducts, suggesting eventual regeneration of these structures. It was suggested, then,

that such temporary structural alterations may induce functional changes in the sebaceous glands and, possibly, sebum production and composition. These proposals remain speculative, and recent studies of sebum production following laser treatment have provided inconsistent results (Bogle *et al.* 2007; Orringer *et al.* 2007; Perez-Maldonado *et al.* 2007). Future studies will need to identify additional factors that may be contributing to the improvement in acne lesions seen with these lasers.

Treatment specifics

As with all light-based treatments, proper patient selection and pretreatment care are important. In the therapy of acne vulgaris, both facial and truncal involvement can be improved with these devices (**23, 24**). Although most studies have documented improvement in inflammatory acne lesions (Bogle *et al.* 2007; Jih *et al.* 2006; Paithankar *et al.* 2002; Wang *et al.* 2006), one study noted a transient reduction in open comedones, suggesting a potential benefit in such a population (Orringer *et al.* 2007). Patients with acne scarring may derive an additional benefit of improvement in their scars, as will be discussed in the next chapter. Although light absorption by epidermal melanin is low throughout the mid-infrared range, it is approximately 1.6 times higher at 1320 nm than at

1540 nm (Mordon *et al.* 2000). It has, therefore, been proposed that the latter wavelength may be slightly safer in darker skin tones. Nevertheless, studies indicate that all mid-infrared lasers may be used safely in all skin types, provided that proper laser parameters and epidermal cooling are utilized (**25, 26**).

Immediately prior to treatment, all makeup needs to be removed to prevent inappropriate absorption of laser energy and subsequent epidermal overheating. The addition of microdermabrasion prior to treatment has not been shown to improve clinical results, at least with the 1450-nm laser (Wang *et al.* 2006). Mild to moderate

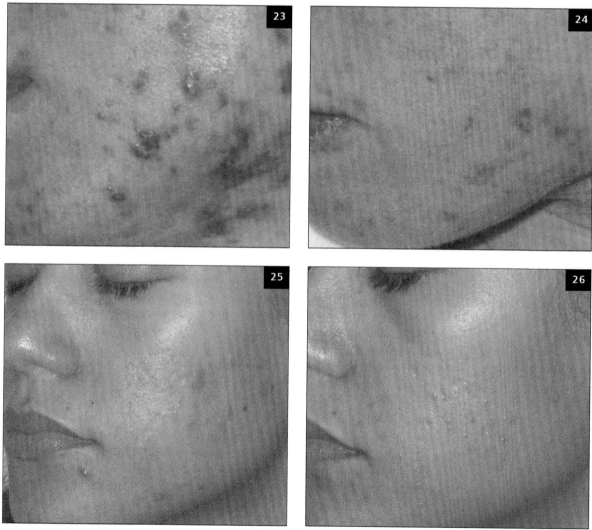

23, 24 Moderate-to-severe acne. 23 Before treatment. **24** Following two sessions with a 1320-nm laser, showing significant improvement in inflammatory lesions.

25, 26 Inflammatory acne in a Hispanic patient. 25 Before treatment. **26** Following three sessions with a 1450-nm laser, demonstrating efficacy and safety in darker skin tones.

pain may be experienced with some devices, especially when higher fluences are utilized, and topical anesthetics may be used based on patient preference. Finally, eye protection needs to be provided in the form of goggles for the practitioner and goggles or gauze for the patient.

Since mid-infrared lasers are able to penetrate deeply into the skin and are nonspecifically absorbed by water, epidermal damage is an important consideration with these devices. Thus, the use of these lasers without their associated cooling devices may result in epidermal necrosis; early 1320-nm lasers equipped only with a prepulse cooling led to an increased risk of blistering, hyperpigmentation, and atrophic scarring (Kelly *et al.* 1999). As a result, all currently-marketed mid-infrared range lasers feature continuous or pulsed epidermal pre-, intra-, and post-treatment cooling. Depending on the device, this is accomplished with either contact cooling using a chilled sapphire window, or liquid cryogen spray, also known as dynamic cooling. In addition, the 1320-nm laser is now also equipped with a thermal sensor to maintain the peak epidermal surface temperature within a defined range, typically 40–45°C (Orringer *et al.* 2007). Considering the importance of epidermal protection, a given cooling system must be tested immediately prior to treatment.

The 1320-nm Nd:YAG laser features a 10 mm spot size, a fixed, 50 msec pulse duration composed of six stacked pulses, and an adjustable fluence. The handpiece contains three portals, including the laser aperture, cryogen spray aperture, and a thermal sensor. In the treatment of acne, the initial fluence is typically set between 12 and 18 J/cm^2. A test firing is performed and fluence is then adjusted to reach the required temperature range, as displayed on the light-emitting diode (LED) screen. Three to four passes are usually undertaken, although no randomized controlled trials have been performed to document greater efficacy of multiple passes in the treatment of acne vulgaris. Pre-, intra-, and postpulse epidermal cooling is achieved with three pulses of a cryogen spray. It should, however, be noted that cryogen may in turn cause cold injury to the epidermis, leading to postinflammatory hyperpigmentation in darkly-pigmented individuals (Kelly *et al.* 1999). Cryogen delivery time should, therefore, be shortened in such cases.

The 1450-nm diode laser features a 4 mm or a 6 mm spot size and an adjustable fluence. The laser pulse consists of four stacked pulses totaling 210 msec, which are interspersed with five cryogen 'spurts' to provide pre-, intra-, and post-treatment epidermal protection. Typical fluences used with this system range from 9 to 14 J/cm^2; fluences higher than 14 J/cm^2 have been found to cause more pain without improved efficacy (Jih *et al.* 2006). In a recent study, a double-pass technique was compared to a stacked-pulse technique, and found to cause less pain and carry a lower risk of hyperpigmentation in darker skin tones (Uebelhoer *et al.* 2007).

The 1540-nm Er:glass laser features a 4 mm spot size, pulse duration of 3.3 msec, and continuous contact cooling using a chilled sapphire tip. This cooling mode results in a generally less painful treatment and more tolerable experience compared to the other mid-infrared devices (Bogle *et al.* 2007). The laser can be used in normal, single-pulse mode, or pulse-train mode with up to 3 pulses/second. Typical fluences range from 8 to 10 J/cm^2 per pulse and a cumulative fluence of up to 60 J/cm^2 in pulse-train mode to prevent epidermal damage (Fournier & Mordon 2005; Lupton & Alster 2001).

Because of their nonablative nature, mid-infrared lasers typically do not require specific postoperative care. Common adverse effects may include mild to moderate transient pain and mild erythema and edema that resolve within 24 hours. Blistering, postinflammatory hyperpigmentation, and, rarely, scarring, are uncommon and may be related to high fluences or excessive cryogen cooling, especially in darker skin types.

Maximum improvement in inflammatory acne requires multiple treatment sessions, typically three to six, administered every 2–4 weeks. Thereafter, periodic maintenance treatments may prolong the overall clinical improvement (Bogle *et al.* 2007), although specific retreatment protocols have not been established. All mid-infrared range lasers appear to have similar clinical efficacy in the treatment of acne; it should, however, be noted that no face-to-face comparisons of the different systems in the treatment of this condition have been published.

PULSED-DYE LASERS

The first randomized controlled trial on the use of pulsed-dye lasers (PDLs) in the treatment of inflammatory acne vulgaris was published in 2003

(Seaton et al. 2003). The study utilized subpurpuric doses, resulting in significant reduction in total and inflammatory acne lesions – 49% in PDL-treated versus 10% in sham laser-treated patients – with a low incidence of adverse effects. A later study, however, failed to show significant improvement in facial acne using the same device, though the study included a large number of dropouts, potentially introducing type 2 errors (Orringer et al. 2004). Two recent studies showed that the improvement following PDL treatment is similar to that achieved with a chemical peel or topical preparations (Karsai et al. 2010, Leheta 2009). Currently-available PDLs usually operate in the 585–595 nm range and may or may not include cooling mechanisms (see Table 10, page 67).

Mechanism of action

A study on the potential mode of action of PDL on inflammatory acne revealed no effect on either *Propionibacterium* acnes counts or sebum excretion rate. The study noted, however, a significant, 5- to 15-fold increase in the expression of transforming growth factor-beta mRNA (Seaton et al. 2006). This cytokine is known to be a potent immunosuppressant, as well as an inhibitor of keratinocyte proliferation, an important factor in the formation of microcomedo (Barnard et al. 1988, Wahl et al. 2004).

Treatment specifics

Prior to treatment, the patient should remove all makeup; proper eye protection has to be worn by the patient and all personnel during treatment, as the emitted wavelength is readily absorbed by the retina and retinal vasculature. Subpurpuric doses can be achieved with either lower fluence or longer pulse duration. In addition, fluences may be further lowered in patients with darker skin tones (Seaton et al. 2003). If available, epidermal cooling may lessen patient discomfort and the risk of dyschromia.

Used at subpurpuric doses, PDL treatments carry a small risk of transient adverse effects, including pain, focal purpura, pruritus, and dyschromia. In addition, a case of ophthalmic herpes zoster following the procedure has also been reported (Clayton & Stables 2005).

Although the original study on the use of PDL in inflammatory acne employed a single treatment, other clinical trials have used other regimens, such as multiple sessions (typically 4–6) administered 2 weeks apart (Choi et al. 2010, Leheta 2009). Thus, the optimal treatment protocol, including the need for maintenance therapy, has yet to be established through further studies.

VISIBLE LIGHT SOURCES AND LIGHT-EMITTING DIODES

Visible light sources were some of the earliest light-based systems used in the treatment of acne vulgaris. Originally, blue light devices were introduced and subsequently gained FDA approval for the treatment of this condition. Later developments in this field include the advent of blue and red LED panels, with the latter device used off-label in the US for this indication.

Mechanism of action

The use of visible light in the treatment of acne vulgaris takes advantage of the intrinsic production of porphyrins, most notably coproporphyrin III and, to a lesser extent, protoporphyrin IX, by *Propionibacterium acnes* (Lee et al. 1978). Activation of porphyrins in the presence of an oxygen molecule produces singlet oxygen species, which is highly reactive and leads to cellular destruction of the bacterium (Arakane et al. 1996; Ashkenazi et al. 2003). The major absorption peaks for coproporphyrin III are 401 nm (maximum) and 548 nm in the visible light spectrum, whereas those for protoporphyrin IX include 410 nm (maximum), 505, 540, 580, and 630 nm (Fritsch et al. 1998; Jope & O'Brien 1945). Although the absorption peak is significantly higher in the blue portion of the light spectrum, the associated wavelength has very limited penetration into the skin. As a result, additional light sources, such as those emitting red light with greater optical penetration depth, have also been used for porphyrin activation and subsequent elimination of *P. acnes* bacteria.

Additional mechanisms may be involved in the improvement of acne vulgaris by visible light sources. Blue light has been found to reduce significantly the expression of interleukin (IL)-1alpha and intercellular adhesion molecule (ICAM)-1 in response to inflammatory cytokines, thus acting as an anti-inflammatory modality (Shnitkind et al. 2006). Likewise, red light at 635 nm has been shown to possess anti-inflammatory qualities, including decreased expression of phospholipase A2 and cyclooxygenase and synthesis of prostaglandin E2 (Lim et al. 2007).

Treatment specifics

Visible light sources can be used in patients of all skin types with facial or truncal inflammatory acne (Kawada *et al.* 2002; Sigurdsson *et al.* 1997) (**27, 28**). In addition, a reduction in the number of comedones has also been noted with the use of blue and combined blue and red light sources (Kawada *et al.* 2002; Papageorgiou *et al.* 2000), although such findings have been inconsistent (Morton *et al.* 2005). Immediately prior to treatment, all makeup is removed and the patient's eyes are protected using goggles or gauze. Treatments are not associated with any significant discomfort, obviating the need for topical anesthesia.

Although the number of clinical trials, both randomized controlled and case series, utilizing visible light sources is fairly large, optimal treatment parameters have not yet been established. Blue light sources on the market today utilize a variety of spectral outputs, such as 405–420 nm (ClearLight, CureLight, Gladstone, NJ, USA), 415 nm (Omnilux blue, Photo Therapeutics Inc., Carlsbad, CA, USA), and 417 nm (BLU-U, DUSA Pharmaceuticals Inc., Wilmington, MA, USA). Red light sources typically vary from 633 (Omnilux revive, Photo Therapeutics Inc., Carlsbad, CA, USA) to 660 nm (various manufacturers). Most regimens utilize twice weekly treatments for 4 weeks, although some studies included daily treatments (Papageorgiou *et al.* 2000), while others alternated exposure to red and blue lights during the twice weekly sessions (Goldberg & Russell 2006). Likewise, optimal exposure times have not been established, with most studies utilizing a 16–20 minute exposure, with shorter exposures of 10 minutes and even as low as 35 seconds also shown to be effective in the treatment of acne (McDaniel *et al.* 2007; Morton *et al.* 2005). These parameters will need to be optimized through additional studies in the future. No specific post-treatment care is required following exposure to visible light devices.

Adverse effects are uncommon with visible light therapy, but may include mild erythema, xerosis, pruritus, acne flare, and headaches (Kawada *et al.* 2002; Morton *et al.* 2005; Papageorgiou *et al.* 2005).

PHOTODYNAMIC THERAPY

Photodynamic therapy (PDT) utilizing 5-aminolevulinic acid (ALA) in combination with a specific blue light source (BLU-U, DUSA Pharmaceuticals Inc., Wilmington, MA, USA) is currently FDA-approved for the treatment of nonhyperkeratotic actinic keratoses on the face and scalp. It also has a long track record of being used off-label for the treatment of acne vulgaris. Additionally, methyl aminolevulinate (MAL), a methyl ester form of ALA, has long been available outside the US for similar indications. It has recently gained FDA approval for the treatment of actinic keratoses, but is not yet available in the US.

Mechanism of action

Although several potential mechanisms of action of PDT in acne vulgaris have been proposed, they have not yet been definitively proven. Hongcharu *et al.* (2000), who pioneered the use of ALA-PDT in the treatment of inflammatory acne, noted decreased sebum production, suppressed bacterial fluorescence, and reduction in the size of the sebaceous glands following treatment. These effects are thought to be the result of the direct action of ALA on the sebocytes and *P. acnes* bacteria; however, additional physiological mechanisms may also be involved, but have yet to be demonstrated.

ALA is part of the porphyrin pathway. When applied topically, ALA accumulates in rapidly-dividing epidermal and dermal cells, as well as within the sebaceous glands (Divaris *et al.* 1990). It is then converted to protoporphyrin IX (PpIX), which is photosensitizing and, as was described in the previous section, leads to the formation of singlet oxygen species upon activation by light. This, in turn, causes cellular membrane disruption and damage to the affected cells, such as to the sebocytes (Kennedy *et al.* 1990). The mechanism appears to be slightly different within *P. acnes* bacteria, as the addition of ALA to the bacterial culture leads to a greater intracellular accumulation of coproporphyrin III, which, as was described in the previous section, also leads to the formation of singlet oxygen species and may lead to bacterial cell death (Ashkenazi *et al.* 2003).

As mentioned before, PpIX has multiple absorption peaks, including 410, 505, 540, 580, and 630 nm (Fritsch *et al.* 1998). Consequently, various lasers and light sources can and have been utilized in PDT for acne vulgaris; however, the longer wavelengths with their enhanced optical penetration depth may be better suited to reach the level of the sebaceous glands within the skin.

Treatment specifics

PDT for the treatment of acne appears to be safe in all skin types, although the published controlled trials and case series have been mostly limited to skin types I–V (Pollock *et al.* 2004). Patients with mild to severe

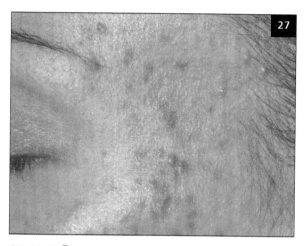

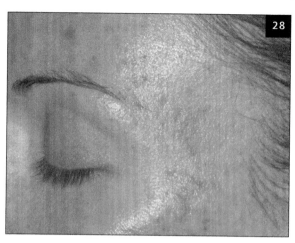

27, 28 **Inflammatory acne. 27** Before treatment. **28** Following two sessions with a combination of a 1320-nm laser and a red light-emitting diode device.

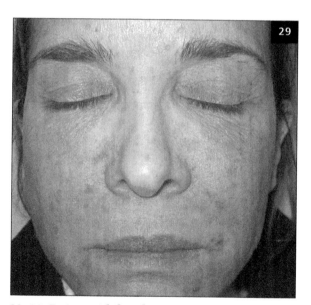

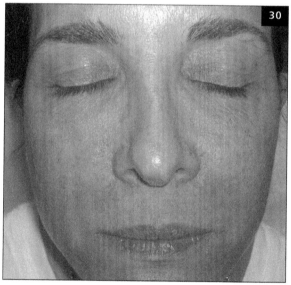

29, 30 **Patient with facial acne. 29** Before treatment. **30** Following three sessions with photodynamic therapy using 5-aminolevulinic acid and a red light-emitting diode device. Notice concomitant improvement in dyschromia associated with photodamaged skin.

inflammatory and cystic acne with facial and truncal involvement are best candidates for this therapy (**29, 30**); however, activation using a long-pulsed pulsed dye laser has recently been shown also to reduce comedonal lesions (Alexiades-Armenakas 2006).

Prior to the application of topical photosensitizers, the treatment area is cleansed and preferably degreased using an acetone scrub or microdermabrasion to increase cutaneous penetration. Recently, fractional resurfacing immediately prior to PDT has been successfully used in photorejuvenation and may theoretically also be of use in the treatment of acne (Ruiz-Rodriguez *et al*. 2007).

The only currently available formulation of ALA in the US is a 20% solution in a single-use applicator (Levulan Kerastick, Dusa Pharmaceuticals, Wilmington, MA,

USA). The solution has to be mixed immediately prior to the application by first applying manual pressure onto the outer glass tubing of the applicator to break the inner ampoules containing the active ingredients, followed by gentle rotation between fingers for 3 minutes to assure adequate mixing. The roll-on applicator tip is then used to apply the chemical evenly over the treatment area.

As was mentioned above, a slightly different photosensitizer, MAL, is currently only available outside the US. It is supplied as a fixed cream formulation containing 16% of the active ingredient (Metvix, PhotoCure ASA/Galderma, Oslo, Norway), which is applied directly over the treatment area. This use is supported by several clinical trials, which indicate that MAL-PDT is effective in the treatment of acne vulgaris (Hörfelt et al. 2006; Wiegell & Wulf 2006a). Moreover, in a direct comparison of ALA-PDT and MAL-PDT, the clinical improvement was found to be similar between the two groups, whereas a greater incidence of erythema, pustular eruptions, and exfoliation was noted with the former technique (Wiegell & Wulf 2006b).

Attempts have been made to optimize incubation times following ALA or MAL application in order to allow adequate penetration while shortening the overall duration of the procedure. While earlier studies typically allowed 3 hours of incubation (Hongcharu et al. 2000; Pollock et al. 2004; Wiegell & Wulf 2006a), more recent evidence suggests that shorter incubations of less than 1 hour–sometimes as little as 15 minutes–may be adequate in the treatment of acne (Alexiades-Armenakas 2006; Goldman & Boyce 2003; Taub 2004).

Multiple lasers and light sources have been used for the activation of topical photosensitizers used in the PDT of acne vulgaris. These include lamp and LED sources of red and blue light, blue light-emitting diode lasers, intense pulsed light, long-pulsed pulsed dye laser, and combined noncoherent light and radiofrequency device (Alexiades-Armenakas 2006; Hongcharu et al. 2000; Pollock et al. 2004; Santos et al. 2005; Taub 2004; Wiegell & Wulf 2006a). Although not currently supported by extensive published data, a recent consensus statement suggested that the best results in the PDT of acne may be achieved with the use of a pulsed dye laser as an activating device (Nestor et al. 2006).

Typically, when using lasers or intense pulsed light (IPL) devices for activation, one or more passes of nonoverlapping pulses are administered over the treatment area. On the other hand, when blue or red lamps and LED devices are utilized, exposure time is usually set at 15–20 minutes. This stems from the original protocol for the treatment of actinic keratoses, which called for 16 minutes and 40 seconds of blue light exposure; however, no studies determining the optimal exposure duration in the treatment of acne have been published.

Following the procedure, a mild cleanser is used to remove any remaining ALA. Alternatively, a source of blue light may be used for 5–8 minutes to deactivate the remaining superficially-localized photosensitizer in a process called photobleaching (Nestor et al. 2006). A broad-spectrum sunblock is then applied and patients are instructed on the complete avoidance of direct exposure to sunlight for 24–48 hours due to an increased risk of a phototoxic reaction.

While most patients tolerate the procedure very well with minimal to no discomfort, short-term adverse effects of PDT in the treatment of acne vulgaris may include mild to severe stinging, burning, or pain during the treatment, transient mild to severe erythema, edema, urticarial wheals, exfoliation, crusting, transient dyschromia, and acneiform pustular eruptions (31–36) (34–36 overleaf). Ice packs and mild topical steroids may improve localized symptomatology, while prolonged incubation times may cause more severe reactions, known as the PDT effect. Additionally, the specific activating systems may carry their own potential adverse effects, such as purpura associated with the use of a pulsed dye laser or incidental hair removal in the areas treated by an intense pulsed light device.

One to four treatment sessions administered in weekly to monthly intervals have most commonly been used in the published studies of PDT in acne vulgaris; however, the optimal treatment schedule and the need for maintenance therapy have not yet been firmly established.

RADIOFREQUENCY DEVICES

Recently, radiofrequency (RF) systems (high-frequency electrical devices that produce alternating current in the range of 0.3–40 MHz) have been successfully tried in a very small number of studies on the treatment of acne.

Mechanism of action

Monopolar RF systems feature a single electrode and a large grounding plate attached at a distance, whereas bipolar RF devices are equipped with two electrodes separated by a short distance. Both types of systems produce electrical flow, either between the two electrodes or between the electrode and the grounding plate. According to Ohm's law, this flow, or electrical current, increases with decreased tissue impedance. As per Joule's law, such current also produces heat in direct proportion to the impedance, and volumetric tissue heating, expressed in J/cm^3, is subsequently achieved.

It has been proposed that such tissue heating may damage sebaceous glands, which may be further aided by the addition of intense pulsed light in some systems. While histological examination of biopsy specimens confirmed a decrease in the size of the sebaceous glands following treatment and demonstrated reduced perifollicular inflammation (Prieto *et al.* 2005), the current knowledge of the potential mechanisms of action of these devices in the treatment of acne vulgaris is very limited.

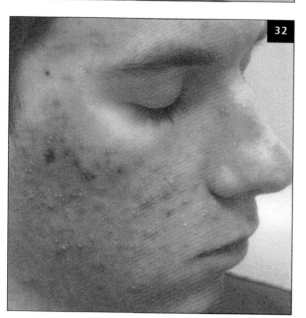

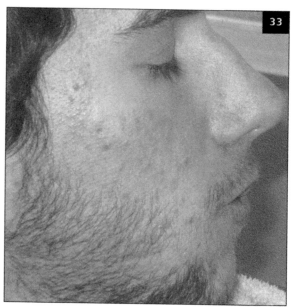

31–33 Patient with inflammatory acne. 31 Before treatment. **32** Patient 2 days after the first photodynamic therapy session using 5-aminolevulinic acid, showing an extensive pustular eruption. **33** Following the resolution of the pustular eruption.

Treatment specifics

In one study, a monopolar device (ThermaCool TC, Thermage Inc., Hayward, CA, USA) equipped with pre-, intra-, and post-treatment cryogen spray cooling was used in conjunction with either a 1 cm^2 or a 0.25 cm^2 electrode tip and energies ranging from 65–103 J/cm^3 (Ruiz-Esparza & Gomez 2003). One to three sessions were used and no adverse effects other than intraoperative mild to moderate pain were noted. Additionally, improvement in acne scars was also noted in some patients.

In a separate study, a bipolar RF device combined with a broadband pulsed light (Aurora AC, Syneron Medical Ltd., Yokneam, Israel) was used in conjunction with contact cooling, optical fluences of 6–10 J/cm^2, and RF energy of 15–20 J/cm^3 (Prieto *et al.* 2005). Patients were treated twice weekly for 4 weeks. No long-term adverse effects were noted, while mild intraoperative discomfort, transient erythema, and three cases of first-degree burns were recorded.

Because of the small number of available studies, the effectiveness of the presented treatment protocols, potential adverse effects, and the duration of clinical effect cannot be properly evaluated at this time. Future studies will need to establish the clinical utility of RF devices in the treatment of acne vulgaris.

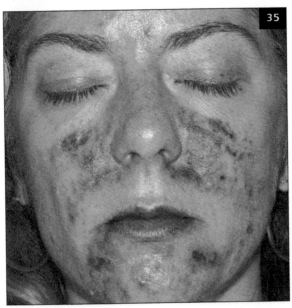

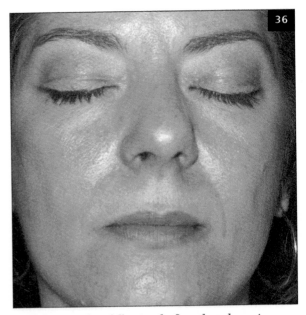

34–36 Patient with inflammatory acne. 34 Before treatment. **35** Patient 4 days following the first photodynamic therapy session using 5-aminolevulinic acid, showing extensive crusting, especially in the areas of coexisting actinic damage. **36** Patient 3 months after three treatment sessions.

4 TREATMENT OF ACNE SCARS

INTRODUCTION

WHILE the previous chapters have dealt with the pathophysiology and treatment of acne vulgaris, this chapter is devoted to the treatment of one of the more unfortunate and yet frequent consequences of the condition, namely scarring. Acne scars can cause significant physical and psychological disability, especially since they, like acne vulgaris, commonly occur during the teenage years.

In recent years, the field of skin resurfacing and rejuvenation has truly blossomed, offering multiple treatment options where few, if any, existed before. Today's treatment modalities offer reliable, predictable, and reproducible improvement in acne scars. This chapter will offer an in-depth look at the various commonly-utilized therapeutic options; however, as the field continues to grow rapidly and expand, the specific equipment and system settings may become outdated or obsolete. Thus, the information is presented with the emphasis on the broad biophysical concepts, as well as on organization and classification of technologies, rather than on the specific treatment parameters for the systems available today.

CLASSIFICATION OF ACNE SCARS

Acne scars vary significantly in their morphology, and a proper classification system is, therefore, important. Many such systems have been developed over the years; however, some are more suitable for descriptive purposes only and cannot be directly and consistently applied to the selection of specific treatment modalities. One of the most therapeutically useful classification schemes has been proposed by Jacob *et al.* (2001). Accordingly, atrophic acne scars are subdivided into ice-pick, rolling, and boxcar varieties. Boxcar scars are then further differentiated into shallow and deep subtypes. On the other end of the spectrum, keloid and hypertrophic scars result from excessive scar tissue formation (37). They occur less frequently than atrophic scars and are more common on the trunk rather than face (Table 3).

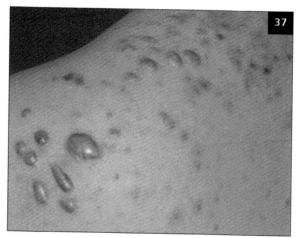

37 **Extensive keloidal scarring** in the presence of active inflammatory acne lesions.

Atrophic	Ice-pick
	Rolling
	Boxcar
	Shallow
	Deep
Hypertrophic	Hypertrophic
	Keloids

(Adapted from Jacob *et al.* [2001].)

Table 3 Classification of acne scars

Ice-pick scars are typically narrow, sharply delineated tracts that taper to a point as they extend to the deep dermis or subcutaneous tissue (**38**). Rolling scars are broad-based skin surface depressions with a resulting undulating appearance (**39**). They are formed by the tethering forces derived from abnormal fibrous adhesions of the dermis to the superficial musculoaponeurotic system. Finally, boxcar scars have a round or oval shape, appear to be 'punched out' with a broad, relatively flat base and vertical edges, and are either less than or greater than 0.5 mm in depth, classified as shallow and deep varieties, respectively (**40**).

As previously mentioned, the differentiation between these subtypes of scars may help to guide the practitioner in the selection of the most appropriate and efficacious therapeutic modality. Since the apex of the ice-pick scars frequently extends beyond the depth of penetration of most resurfacing tools, a punch excision is usually undertaken prior to resurfacing. Tethering forces that account for the appearance of rolling scars need to be released using subcision in order to achieve the best clinical results. The relatively normal, but depressed, skin at the base of deep boxcar scars may be properly repositioned using punch elevation techniques. Finally, the shallow variety of boxcar scars and similarly-appearing varicella scars may be improved with the help of various resurfacing modalities without any pretreatment. Since patients may exhibit many of these varieties of scars simultaneously, multiple techniques are frequently combined. These techniques will now be examined in-depth.

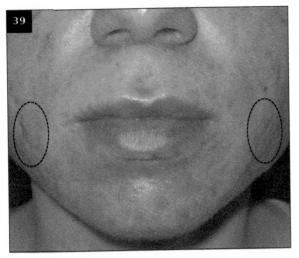

38 Numerous ice-pick acne scars.

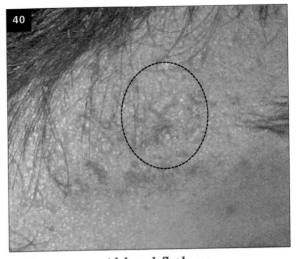

39 Rolling-type acne scars.

40 Boxcar scars with broad, flat bases.

SURGICAL OPTIONS: PUNCH EXCISION, SUBCISION, PUNCH ELEVATION

Although other techniques, such as punch grafting and dermal planing have been utilized for the correction of scars, punch excision, subcision, and punch elevation are the most commonly utilized surgical treatment modalities and will be discussed here.

Punch excision is best reserved for ice-pick scars, as well as for some narrow, deep boxcar scars. Following local infiltrative anesthesia, an excision down to fat is performed using a disposable round punch tool. The diameter of the punch tool should match the diameter of the scar, including the walls. If the scar measures more than 4 mm in diameter, an elliptical excision may be preferred to a punch excision in order to avoid dog-ear formation. The scar is then removed, and the wound is repaired in a usual, everted manner using a single suture (**41–43**). A standard dressing, typically consisting of an antibiotic ointment and a bandage, is then applied to the wound. Additional scars may be excised on the same day, as long as they are spaced at least 5 mm apart to prevent undue tension on the wound. The patient is then instructed on local wound care. The sutures are removed 5–7 days later, thus preventing the appearance of track marks. Resurfacing, as described later in this chapter, may then be used 4–6 weeks later to achieve an even less conspicuous appearance of the scars.

The technique of subcision, or subcutaneous incision, was first developed by Orentreich & Orentreich (1995). This procedure is most useful

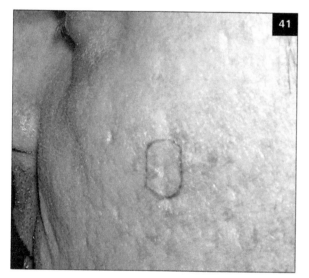

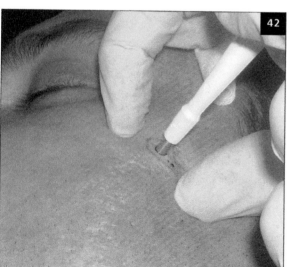

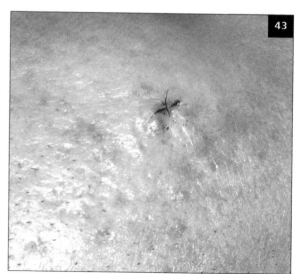

41–43 **Punch excision of an ice-pick acne scar. 41** Before treatment. **42** Excision using a disposable punch tool. **43** Following closure with a suture.

for rolling scars, which result from fibrous adhesions of dermis to deeper structures (**44**). In the process, such adhesions are released, allowing for the otherwise relatively normal skin to assume a more relaxed, nontethered appearance. A triangularly-shaped 18-gauge NoKor Admix needle (Becton, Dickinson and Company, Franklin Lakes, NJ, USA) may be used for the procedure (**45**) (Alam *et al.* 2005). The needle is first attached to a 1 ml or 3 ml empty syringe, and the position of the slanted cutting edge of the needle is noted in relation to the markings on the syringe. Alternatively, a corresponding mark may be placed on the syringe using a surgical marker. Once the needle is inserted under the skin, this will serve to guide the needle in the proper direction of movement. Infiltrative anesthesia is then achieved, and the needle is introduced horizontally near the edge of the scarred area. Once the needle reaches the subcutaneous fat, the syringe is used as a handle to locate and, with a gentle back and forth motion, to cut the fibrous bands. As previously mentioned, care must be exercised at all times to ensure that the cutting edge of the needle is horizontal—that is, parallel to the skin surface—and facing the adhesions. The needle is then withdrawn and the wound is covered with an antibiotic ointment. No suturing of the wound is necessary. Finally, a pressure dressing is applied over the entire undermined area to reduce the risk of bleeding and hematoma formation. In addition to bruising and rare infection and bleeding, adverse effects may also include nodule formation from excessive fibroplasia, which frequently resolved spontaneously or may be treated with an intralesional steroid injection. Multiple sessions of subcision are sometimes necessary. In addition, other techniques, such as filler material injections or laser resurfacing, may be used in conjunction with this procedure to achieve the best clinical results.

Punch elevation works best for deep boxcar acne and varicella scars, where the walls extend vertically down to the relatively normal base. Following local infiltrative anesthesia, a disposable punch tool, selected to match exactly the diameter of the scar, is used to incise the skin to the level of subcutaneous fat (**46**). The resulting tissue is then elevated to just above the level of the surrounding skin to account for subsequent retraction. Sutures, Steri-Strips (3M, St. Paul, MN, USA), or a 2-octyl cyanoacrylate skin adhesive (Dermabond, Ethicon, Inc., Sommerville, NJ, USA) is then used to affix the tissue in place (Jacob *et al.* 2001). An antibiotic

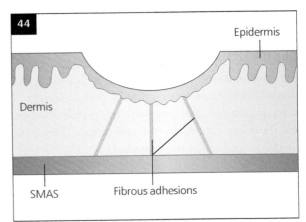

44 A schematic drawing of tethering forces involved in the formation of rolling-type acne scars. SMAS: superficial musculoaponeurotic system.

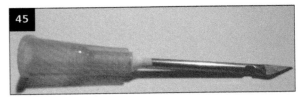

45 An admix needle.

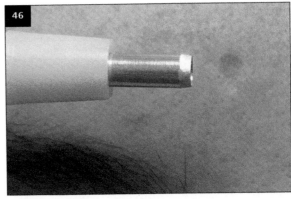

46 Selection of a properly-sized disposable punch tool for punch elevation of a boxcar scar.

ointment and a nonstick dressing are applied to the wound and the patient is instructed on the proper gentle wound care. If sutures are utilized, they are removed after 5–7 days, while resurfacing may be considered after an additional 4–6 weeks.

DERMAROLLER

Dermaroller, also known as microneedling or percutaneous collagen induction therapy, has been gaining popularity for the treatment of scars due to the ease of use, low incidence of adverse effects, and low cost. Though large prospective studies are lacking, significant retrospective and smaller prospective studies suggest efficacy in the improvement of acne scarring (Aust et al. 2008, Majid 2009).

A typical dermaroller is a single-use plastic cylindrical roller studded with microneedles ranging from 0.5 to 3 mm in length and 0.1 mm in diameter. In addition, smaller versions, known as dermastamps, have also been introduced for smaller scars. Using the dermaroller 15 times over the same area has been shown to result in approximately 250 microperforations per cm^2. This, in turn, leads to new collagen and elastic fiber deposition in the subsequent wound healing process. Thickened epidermis has also been demonstrated following this procedure (Aust et al. 2008). Studies suggest good to excellent improvement, especially in mild-to-moderate rolling and boxcar scars (Majid 2009) and significant objective improvement using both the Vancouver Scar Scale and the Patient and Observer Scar Assessment Scale (Aust et al. 2008).

Prior to treatment, an anesthetic cream is applied to the skin. Rolling is then performed 15 to 20 times in vertical, horizontal, and diagonal directions. Deep scars should be stretched to allow the needles to penetrate the base of the scar. Immediately following the procedure, damp gauze or pads are applied to the area to absorb serous oozing and to facilitate healing.

Adverse effects may include erythema, typically lasting 2–3 days, mild-to-moderate edema and bruising for approximately 4–7 days, and crusting for 1–2 days. Cases of herpes simplex infection and rare transient postinflammatory hyperpigmentation have been reported following microneedling (Majid 2009). Three to four sessions, performed every 4–6 weeks, are typically required to achieve the best clinical results.

CHEMICAL RECONSTRUCTION OF SKIN SCARS (CROSS) TECHNIQUE

A novel technique of focal chemical treatment of acne scars has been introduced by Lee et al. (2002). This modality, called chemical reconstruction of skin scars (CROSS) method by the original authors, can be very effective in the improvement of the various types of deep acne scars.

In the process, a high-concentration trichloroacetic acid (TCA), usually between 85% and 100%, is applied focally to the scars. When applied to the skin, lower concentrations of TCA, up to 35%, are known to cause protein precipitation, manifesting as 'frosting' and resulting in coagulative necrosis of the epidermis and collagen degradation down to the upper reticular dermis (Brodland et al. 1989; Brody 1989; Butler et al. 2001; Dailey et al. 1998; El-Domyati et al. 2004). Subsequent collagen remodeling and reorganization of dermal structural elements as a result of wound repair processes then lead to an augmentation of dermal volume (Stegman 1982). Although chemical peeling using high-concentration TCA may lead to scarring and is, therefore, strongly discouraged, focal application of the chemical localized to deep acne scars appears to be safe and effective, even in darker skin types (Lee et al. 2002; Yug et al. 2006). This is likely the result of epidermal sparing, including that of adnexal structures, in the surrounding, untreated skin. Clinically, a gradual elevation of the scar is observed over several months, while histological evidence of immediate coagulative necrosis with subsequent increased epidermal and dermal thickness, increased collagen content, and reorganization of abnormal elastic fibers has been demonstrated (Cho et al. 2006; Yug et al. 2006).

Prior to treatment, the affected skin is thoroughly cleansed with alcohol or acetone. No anesthesia is typically necessary, as the mild focal burning or stinging sensation is well tolerated by most patients. The chemical is then applied to the base of the scar using firm pressure with a sharpened wooden applicator with a slightly dulled tip until white frosting is observed, typically around 10 seconds. The procedure is then repeated to cover the entire depressed area. No post-treatment neutralization of TCA is needed, but a topical antibiotic ointment is applied to the wound without an occlusive dressing (Lee et al. 2002). Patients are then instructed on local wound care, typically consisting of mild cleansing and the application of an antibiotic ointment, as well as on strict sun protection.

It is important to discuss the expected postoperative appearance of the treated areas, with a typical progression of colors from white to gray to brown-black and subsequent desquamation. Common adverse effects of the procedure include mild erythema lasting up to 8 weeks, transient postinflammatory hyperpigmentation lasting up to 6 weeks, and mild acneiform eruptions. On the other hand, no serious or long-term complications, such as persistent dyschromia, herpetic reactivation, or scarring, have been noted in studies. Of note, two patients with a history of recent oral isotretinoin intake were treated in one of the studies without subsequent development of keloids (Lee *et al*. 2002), although the small number of patients precludes a definitive statement on this matter. Multiple treatment sessions (usually three to six) are often necessary in order to achieve the best clinical improvement. The procedure may be repeated every 4–6 weeks.

INJECTABLES IN THE TREATMENT OF ATROPHIC ACNE SCARS

Soft tissue fillers have long been used for a multitude of cosmetic applications, most notably rhytid correction and facial contouring and augmentation (Klein 2006; Lupo 2006; Matarasso 2006; Monheit & Coleman 2006; Tzikas 2008). Various injectable filler materials have also been used for the correction of atrophic acne scars, both singly or in conjunction with other treatment modalities discussed in this chapter (**47,48**) (Barnett & Barnett 2005; Beer 2007; Coleman 2006; Goldberg *et al*. 2006; Varnavides *et al*. 1987). It should, however, be noted that the use of all injectable fillers for the improvement of acne scars is considered off-label in the US.

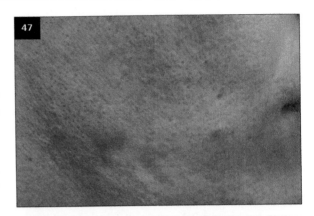

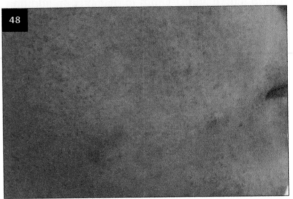

47, 48 **Acne scars. 47** Before treatment. **48** After two treatments with a dermal filler.

Currently-available fillers may be divided into permanent and temporary ones. Examples of permanent fillers include silicone oil (Silikon 1000, Alcon, Inc., Hünenberg, Switzerland), autologous fat transfer, polymethylmethacrylate (ArteFill, Artes Medical, Inc., San Diego, CA, USA), as well as a polyacrylamide hydrogel filler (Aquamid, Contura International A/S, Soeborg, Denmark) currently available outside the US. Examples of materials used in temporary fillers include collagen (Cosmoderm and Cosmoplast, Allergan, Inc., Irvine, CA, USA; Evolence, ColBar LifeScience Ltd., Herzlyia, Israel), hyaluronic acid (Restylane and Perlane, Medicis Aesthetics Inc., Scottsdale, AZ, USA; Juvederm Ultra and Ultra Plus, Allergan, Inc., Irvine, CA, USA), calcium hydroxylapatite (Radiesse, BioForm Medical, San Mateo, CA, USA), and poly-L-lactic acid (Sculptra or New-Fill, Dermik Laboratories, Berwyn, PA, USA).

Prior to treatment, the practitioner should be thoroughly familiar with the specific filler selected for this application, including its proper placement, duration of action, and potential complications and adverse effects. These are discussed at length in numerous review articles and will not be covered in this section, as new products are constantly being developed.

Proper patient selection is of the utmost importance, as ice-pick scars tend to resist treatment with injectable fillers. Rolling acne scars may require subcision to release adhesions prior to injection, while boxcar scars tend to fare the best with this approach. A useful technique is the 'pinch test', in which the scar is pinched between the thumb and the index finger. Partial correction indicates a possibly successful outcome, whereas the absence of correction or deepening of the scar secondary to tethering from the underlying adhesions indicates a likely failure of this type of therapy. In addition, active inflammatory or infectious condition at the intended treatment site is a contraindication to filler placement, while the use of anticoagulative agents increases the risk of bruising.

Multiple-angle, high-quality photographs should be obtained prior to treatment, and tangential lighting may be used to document the depth of the scars. If required, anesthesia may be achieved with topical anesthetic agents or with nerve blocks. Infiltrative anesthesia should be avoided to prevent distortion of the treatment area. The filler is then placed underneath each acne scar at the proper depth for the individual product. For larger scars, serial puncture, linear threading, and fanning techniques, or a combination thereof, may be used to achieve the best correction. Depending on the specific injectable product, under- or over-correction may sometimes be necessary.

Ice-packs can be utilized postoperatively to decrease swelling and bruising. If needed, additional treatment sessions may be performed in 2–4 weeks.

LASERS AND LASER-LIKE DEVICES: TRADITIONAL ABLATIVE RESURFACING

Traditional ablative devices used in the resurfacing of acne scars include carbon dioxide (CO_2, multiple models) and erbium:yttrium–aluminum–garnet (Er:YAG, multiple models) lasers. More recently, an erbium:yttrium–scandium–gallium–garnet (Er:YSGG) laser, emitting light at 2790 nm and with the depth of ablation between those of CO_2 and Er:YAG lasers, has been added to the lineup of ablative lasers, though its specific role in the treatment of acne scars will need to be established in future studies (Ross *et al.* 2009). In addition, a plasma skin resurfacing[3] device (Energist NA, Nyack, NY, USA) (ablative at higher energy levels) has also received FDA clearance for this indication.

Skin ablation results from the evaporation of water and subsequent tissue desiccation. Both the CO_2 and Er:YAG lasers utilize specific absorptive properties of the water molecule, whereas the plasma skin resurfacing device delivers nonspecific thermal energy to the epidermis, which is then propagated to the upper dermis. Originally, the improvement associated with cutaneous resurfacing was mainly attributed to the ablation of the superficial skin layers. Today, however, thermal diffusion to the dermis, also known as residual thermal damage, with the resulting collagen denaturation and subsequent wound remodeling are thought to form the basis for such an improvement.

Collagen fibril is a right-handed helix with three polypeptide chains held together by hydrogen bonds. When collagen is heated, these bonds rupture, leading to a random-coil configuration (Nagy *et al.* 1974; Verzar & Nagy 1970). Thermal denaturation thus results in irreversible shortening and thickening of the collagen fibrils, which later serve as a template for neocollagenesis. The subsequent process of wound remodeling leads to the deposition of new fetal-type collagen type III, later to be replaced by the more mature collagen type I, as well as neoelastogenesis and the repair of the three-dimensional elastic fiber network (Tsukahara *et al.* 2001). In fact, the dermis continues to exhibit progressively increasing collagen content with horizontal alignment of fibers, still evident 12–18 months following resurfacing with a CO_2 laser (Rosenberg *et al.* 1999; Walia & Alster 1999a).

Proper patient selection and pretreatment care are critical to the success of the procedure. Thus, ablative resurfacing, especially in association with the more aggressive treatment parameters, should be reserved for deeper atrophic scars, whereas patients with milder scarring may benefit sufficiently from nonablative or fractional devices, as described in subsequent sections. The ideal candidate for ablative laser resurfacing has Fitzpatrick skin type I–III, expresses realistic expectations about the procedure, and is able to follow strict wound care instructions. A review of past medical history should be performed with the emphasis on keloidal scar formation, as well as conditions predisposing to infections or poor wound healing. Although a history of recent oral isotretinoin intake in the preceding 6 months is considered by some practitioners to increase the risk of keloidal scarring following ablative resurfacing procedures (Katz & MacFarlane 1994; Rubenstein *et al.* 1986; Zachariae 1988), other studies appear to refute such evidence (Dzubow & Miller 1987).

A recent study on the use of multiple topical products, including glycolic acid, hydroquinone, and tretinoin, prior to ablative resurfacing showed no reduction in the incidence of postoperative hyperpigmentation (West & Alster 1999). Antibiotic prophylaxis prior to ablative resurfacing, potentially of most importance with a CO_2 laser, is controversial, as various regimens have been proposed but not validated (Conn & Nanda 2000; Friedman & Geronemus 2000; Gaspar *et al.* 2001; Manuskiatti *et al.* 1999; Ross *et al.* 1998; Walia & Alster 1999b). In addition, such use of antibiotics may lead to the emergence of resistant bacterial strains. The use of antiviral prophylaxis, however, is critical to decrease the incidence of herpetic outbreaks and dissemination (Monheit 1995). It is typically initiated 2–5 days prior to ablative resurfacing and is continued until full regeneration of the stratum corneum.

Preoperative anesthesia for ablative resurfacing using an Er:YAG laser or the plasma skin resurfacing device is typically achieved with topical anesthetic agents or nerve blocks. On the other hand, CO_2 laser resurfacing usually requires intravenous sedation or general anesthesia. Finally, an operational plume evacuator is mandatory for all ablative resurfacing procedures (Garden *et al.* 2002). Ablative resurfacing is then performed over the entire affected cosmetic units or, more frequently, over the entire face to avoid the appearance of the lines of demarcation following the healing phase.

With the CO_2 laser, the entire epidermis is usually ablated with the first pass of nonoverlapping pulses. In total, one to three passes may be undertaken, depending on the depth and the severity of acne scarring. Unless only a single pass is performed, the desiccated debris is wiped off using saline-soaked gauze between the passes (Alster & West 1996; Walia & Alster 1999a).

When using Er:YAG lasers, 2–4 μm of tissue depth are predictably ablated for each J/cm^2 of fluence. In this manner, the total depth of ablation can be accurately controlled by varying fluence and the number of passes. The desiccated debris does not need to be wiped off after each pass. If needed, pulses may be partially overlapped (Jeong & Kye 2001; Tanzi & Alster 2003a).

While a single pass using lower energy of 1–2 J may be sufficient when treating mild acne scarring with the plasma skin resurfacing device, higher energy settings of 3–4 J may utilized in more severe cases. In such instances, one to two passes consisting of nonoverlapping pulses may be performed, with the desiccated debris left intact between passes and after the final pass to serve as a biological wound dressing (Gonzalez *et al.* 2008).

Postoperative care following ablative resurfacing is generally subdivided into closed and open methods. The closed method utilizes a variety of dressings, such as hydrogels, foams, and polymer films, in order to provide a moist protective environment with a low oxygen surface tension to facilitate wound healing. The open method consists of frequent applications of occlusive petrolatum-based or similar ointments. While the open method is usually sufficient following treatment with a plasma skin resurfacing device, the closed method or a combination of these methods may be utilized after a CO_2 and Er:YAG laser resurfacing.

While clearly effective, treatment of acne scars with ablative devices, especially at the more aggressive settings, is fraught with potential adverse effects. Erythema occurs in all treated patients and lasts 1–9

months with a CO_2 laser, 4–12 weeks with an Er:YAG laser, and 3–14 days with the plasma device. Edema, crusting, and pruritus are common in the immediate postoperative period. Various infections, including bacterial, mycobacterial, fungal, and viral, have been reported following ablative procedures with the CO_2 and Er:YAG lasers and, as mentioned previously, the use of pretreatment antiherpetic prophylaxis is mandatory. Transient postinflammatory hyperpigmentation typically occurs in darker skin tones (skin types III and above) (Kilmer *et al.* 2007; Nanni & Alster 1998; Tanzi & Alster 2003b; Teikemeier & Goldberg 1997). Delayed-onset permanent hypopigmentation, on the other hand, occurs in individuals with skin types I and II, with only rare reports in skin type III. This unfortunate complication may start as late as 1 year following ablative resurfacing and has been noted to occur in as many as 16% of patients with fair complexion treated with the CO_2 laser, and approximately 4% of those treated with the Er:YAG laser (Bernstein *et al.* 1997; Weinstein 1999; Zachary 2000). So far, this complication has not been documented with the plasma device (Bogle *et al.* 2007; Kilmer *et al.* 2007). The incidence of contact dermatitis following ablative resurfacing may be reduced with consistent hypoallergenic wound care regimens and the avoidance of makeup and other products until full re-epithelialization. Acne and milia formation is fairly common and may be treated with standard acne therapies. Finally, permanent scarring seldom occurs with the more aggressive therapies, such as the CO_2 laser resurfacing, but may be related to postoperative infections or improper treatment techniques (Nanni & Alster 1998).

LASERS AND LASER-LIKE DEVICES: TRADITIONAL NONABLATIVE RESURFACING

Nonablative resurfacing, also known as dermal or subsurface resurfacing, has been developed in response to the prolonged recovery time and the high incidence of adverse effects associated with the ablative modalities. In the treatment of acne scarring, their mechanism of action appears to be similar to that of the ablative lasers, with selective heating of upper dermal water and subsequent collagen denaturation and dermal remodeling with epidermal preservation afforded by a variety of cooling devices (Tanzi & Alster 2004). Additionally, various matrix modulators, such as matrix metalloproteinases

(MMPs), may be modified by these treatments and may contribute to the clinical improvement seen with these lasers (Oh *et al.* 2007; Orringer *et al.* 2005). The same mid-infrared lasers discussed in the previous chapter in the context of the treatment of active acne vulgaris can also be used for nonablative resurfacing of acne scars (*Table 4 overleaf*) (Rogachefsky *et al.* 2003; Tanzi & Alster 2004).

Patient selection, preoperative care, treatment parameters, and adverse effects are essentially identical to those explored at length in the previous chapter. The reader is invited to review pertinent information from that chapter at this time. Although significantly less effective than their ablative counterparts at improving acne scars, the nonablative devices are associated with no or very brief downtime and few, if any, adverse effects (**49, 50**). Relative effectiveness of the nonablative lasers in the improvement of acne scars appears to be similar; however, only one comparative study has so far been performed. That study demonstrated better clinical results with the 1450-nm laser as compared to the 1320-nm laser; however, somewhat suboptimal parameters were utilized with the latter device (Tanzi & Alster 2004)

LASERS AND LASER-LIKE DEVICES: FRACTIONAL RESURFACING

The concept of fractional photothermolysis arose from the perceived need to combine the unequivocal effectiveness of ablative systems with the tolerability and rapid recovery associated with the nonablative lasers.

Since the introduction of the first laser based on fractional delivery of the laser beam, multiple systems have now been developed and utilized in the treatment of acne scars (*Table 5*). Similar to traditional lasers, they are sometimes subdivided into ablative and nonablative fractional systems. It should, however, be noted that this distinction is somewhat arbitrarily based on the amount of epidermal damage, since at least some degree of ablation occurs with all of these systems.

The first commercially-available system (Fraxel SR750, Solta Medical, Inc., Hayward, CA, USA) utilized a 1550 nm erbium-doped fiber laser to form arrays of columns of thermal damage, also known as microscopic treatment zones (MTZs). The newest generation of this system (Fraxel SR1500 or re:store, Solta Medical, Inc., Hayward, CA, USA) is able to penetrate deeper into the dermis and does not require the application of blue dye to the treatment area. Laser light emitted by these systems is mainly absorbed by water, with subsequent heat propagation within the dermis, collagen denaturation, and wound remodeling, which is then thought to account for the clinical improvement in acne scars (Rahman *et al.* 2006). Unlike traditional lasers, however, resurfacing occurs in columnar, or vertical, manner, thus leaving intact tissue immediately surrounding each MTZ and facilitating subsequent healing (Laubach *et al.* 2006; Manstein *et al.* 2004).

Nonablative fractional laser resurfacing can be utilized in patients of all skin types, although special considerations in darker skin tones will be discussed

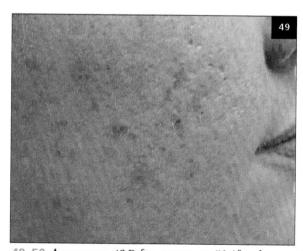
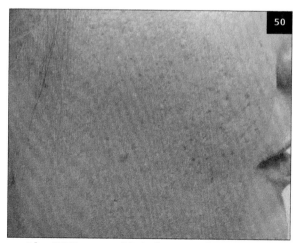

49, 50 **Acne scars. 49** Before treatment. **50** After three sessions with a 1320-nm nonablative laser resurfacing.

below. As with ablative resurfacing, a history of recent isotretinoin intake is considered by some practitioners to be a contraindication to the procedure; however, no direct evidence of increased incidence of keloidal scarring with this device has so far been documented. Oral antiviral prophylaxis is instituted 2–5 days prior to the procedure in patients with prior history of herpes labialis, especially if periorificial resurfacing is planned.

Preoperative anesthesia for nonablative fractional resurfacing is typically achieved with topical anesthetic agents. All makeup is removed prior to the procedure and a petroleum-based ointment may be applied to facilitate handpiece gliding. As the handpiece is moved over the treatment area, the delivery of columns of photothermolysis is automatically adjusted, based on the velocity of such movement. If the velocity is excessive, a higher-pitched sound is used to notify the practitioner. Unlike its ablative counterpart, fractional resurfacing may be limited to the problem areas alone without the risk of formation of the lines of demarcation.

The percentage of treated area directly affected by the laser beam is related to the total MTZ density—a product of MTZ density per pass and the total number of passes. For the improvement of acne scars, a typical recommended total MTZ density is 1000–2000 per cm^2 per treatment session (Alster et al. 2007; Hasegawa et al. 2006). On the other hand, energy level is selected based on the desired depth of penetration, corresponding to the depth of the acne scars. Patient discomfort may, however, be a limiting factor; thus, the width of the MTZ column automatically increases with higher energy levels. In addition, air cooling, such as that afforded by the Cryo5 device (Zimmer Elektromedizin GmbH, Neu-Ulm, Germany), may lead to greater patient tolerability (Fisher et al. 2005).

Postoperative wound care consists of the use of petrolatum-based ointments or bland moisturizers until complete resolution of epidermal desquamation, with subsequent strict sun protection, especially important in darker skinned individuals. Multiple treatment sessions, usually three to five, are needed for the best cosmetic improvement and may be administered every 1–4 weeks. As with other resurfacing modalities, patients should be notified of the delayed onset of improvement in acne scars, owing to the gradual nature of postprocedural dermal remodeling.

Common adverse effects following nonablative fractional photothermolysis include transient erythema, typically lasting 2–3 days, and mild edema for 1–2 days. Flaking and bronzing secondary to transepidermal extrusion of concentrated melanin usually begin several days following the procedure and resolve by 1–2 weeks (Alster et al. 2007; Manstein et al. 2004). Transient postinflammatory hyperpigmentation is common in individuals with darker skin tones. Recent studies suggest, however, that, while both the density and energy of fractionated laser beam may be important, the total MTZ density appears to be a greater determinant of this adverse effect. Epidermal air cooling may also decrease the incidence of postprocedural dyschromia (Chan et al. 2007). No long-term or permanent adverse effects, such as delayed-onset hypopigmentation or scarring, have so far been reported with nonablative fractional resurfacing.

With the success of fractional technology, additional devices have since been developed. Two systems, StarLux with a Lux1540 fractional handpiece (Palomar Medical Technologies, Inc., Burlington, MA, USA) and Affirm (Cynosure, Inc., Westford, MA, USA), feature handpiece tips with fixed-pattern fractionation of the laser beam, as well as built-in contact cooling. As well, the latter system emits sequential pulses of light with wavelengths of 1440 nm and 1320 nm, allowing the use of lower fluences with each of the two wavelengths. Both of these fractional systems may be used off-label for the treatment of acne scarring; however, future prospective studies will need to confirm their utility for this indication.

Fractional technology has now also been implemented with other lasers, such as CO_2, Er:YAG, and Er:YSGG (Table 5). These so-called 'ablative fractional lasers' may offer greater improvement compared to the previously introduced fractional systems, but are also associated with greater downtime and, potentially, a greater incidence of adverse effects. Although topical anesthesia may be sufficient for some patients, nerve blocks and oral anxiolytics may be required in others prior to such treatments, especially at higher energy settings. Following ablative fractional resurfacing, strict wound care consisting of the aforementioned open method is essential to maintain epidermal hydration and to facilitate healing. Mild to moderate postoperative erythema may last for 2–4 weeks and occasionally for up to 3 months. Transient edema, petechiae, crusting, and oozing

Name	Manufacturer	Wavelength (nm)	Cooling
CoolTouch CT3	CoolTouch	1320	Cryogen
ThermaScan	Sciton	1319	Contact
SmoothBeam	Candela	1450	Cryogen
Aramis	Quantel Derma	1540	Contact

Table 4 Examples of commercially-available mid-infrared lasers

Type	Name	Manufacturer	Wavelength (nm)	Fractionation pattern	Cooling
Nonablative	Fraxel SR750	Solta Medical	1550	Computer-generated (based on handpiece movement)	None
	Fraxel SR1500 (re:store)	Solta Medical	1550	Computer-generated (based on handpiece movement)	None
	StarLux 500 with Lux1540 Fractional handpiece	Palomar	1540	Fixed-array	Cryogen (only with 10 mm tip)
	Affirm	Cynosure	1440, 1320	Fixed-array	Chilled air
Ablative	Fraxel re:pair	Solta Medical	10600	Computer-generated (based on handpiece movement)	None
	UltraPulse Encore with ActiveFX handpiece	Lumenis	10600	Computer-generated (variable)	None
	with DeepFX handpiece				
	ProFractional	Sciton	2940	Computer-generated (variable)	None
	StarLux 500 with Lux2940 Fractional handpiece	Palomar	2940	Computer-generated (variable)	None
	Burane XL	Quantel Derma	2940	Computer-generated (variable)	None
	Pearl Fractional	Cutera	2790	Computer-generated (variable)	None

Table 5 Examples of commercially-available fractional lasers

also occur in the majority of patients, typically resolving by 1–4 weeks. Although postinflammatory hyperpigmentation has been documented with fractional CO_2 laser resurfacing, delayed-onset hypopigmentation seen with the traditional CO_2 devices has not been reported to date (Chapas *et al*. 2008). It is important to note, however, that the incidence of this and other potential complications will be better ascertained only after prolonged experience with these devices.

Following on the success of laser fractionation, numerous other systems (currently available or in the late stages of testing) will undoubtedly be studied for acne scarring in the next few years. In the end, these developments will likely provide patients with more options and effective clinical improvement of their scars.

TREATMENT OF KELOID AND HYPERTROPHIC ACNE SCARS

Keloid and hypertrophic scars resulting from acne are similar to other types of keloid scarring occurring from other inciting factors, such as surgery, trauma, and inflammation. As previously mentioned, this type of acne scarring is more common on the trunk rather than the face and also occurs more frequently in patients with darker skin tones. As opposed to keloids, hypertrophic scars never outgrow the margins of the original wound and may regress over time.

Although the exact pathophysiology of keloid scarring has not been fully elucidated, abnormal healing response with persistent collagen production, an unbalanced production of collagen type I versus type III, and anomalous expression of a variety of growth factors, growth factor receptors, and regulators of extracellular matrix have been implicated in its formation (Abergel et al. 1985, Fujiwara et al. 2005, Lee et al. 1991, Ong et al. 2007, Uitto et al. 1985, Wolfram et al. 2009, Younai et al. 1996).

Treatment of keloid and hypertrophic acne scarring is similar to that of other types of excessive scarring and most commonly includes intralesional steroids, occlusion, surgical excision, cryosurgery, pulsed-dye laser, and radiation.

Intralesional injections are typically performed using triamcinolone, though hydrocortisone, methyl-prednisolone, and dexamethasone are also utilized for this purpose. Corticosteroids are thought to work by decreasing collagen synthesis and inhibiting fibroblast proliferation (Carroll et al. 2002, Kauh et al. 1997). Although recurrence rates could be unpredictable with this therapy, efficacy rates significantly increase when it is combined with excision or cryotherapy (Sharma et al. 2007, Yosipovitch et al. 2001). Adverse effects of corticosteroids include epidermal or fat atrophy, the development of telangiectasias, and hypopigmentation.

Silicone gel sheets have long been used for the treatment of keloid scars and appear to be especially effective after surgical excision. The exact mechanism of action for this modality is unknown. Although these dressings have to be applied for at least 12 hours daily for several months, their minimal adverse effect profile makes them an appealing option for some patients (Gold et al. 2001).

Performed by itself, surgical excision or shave removal carries an extremely high risk of recurrence, ranging from 50 to 100%, often leading to even larger keloids (Wolfram et al. 2009). Excision is, thus, commonly combined with other techniques, such as intralesional steroid injection or topical imiquimod cream. The latter is a topical immune modulator that increases local production of interferon-alpha, thought be have antifibrotic action (Jacob et al. 2003).

Cryotherapy has been shown to be effective in the treatment of keloids and is thought to alter fibroblast differentiation and activity (Dalkowski et al. 2003). As previously mentioned, this modality can also be combined with intralesional corticosteroid injections. The most common adverse effects include dyschromia and atrophic scarring.

Pulsed-dye lasers are also commonly used for keloids (Alster 1994). Laser light has been shown to downregulate the expression of tumor growth factor-beta 1, upregulate matrix metalloproteinase-13, and to trigger the mitogen-activated protein kinases pathway (Kuo et al. 2005, Kuo et al. 2007). This results in reduced fibroblast proliferation and collagen type III deposition (Kuo et al. 2004).

Finally, radiation therapy is usually reserved for the most treatment-resistant keloids. It is very effective at penetrating into the dermis and causing decreased fibroblast proliferation (Ogawa et al. 2007). However, in addition to dyschromia, its adverse effect profile includes radiation dermatitis and possible carcinogenesis, though the latter risk appears to be low (Botwood et al. 1999, Ogawa et al. 2009).

Although multiple treatment options for keloids and hypertrophic acne scarring exist today, current therapeutic modalities are often insufficient to cause full regression when used alone. Combination therapies, as well as future developments in the field, should provide patients with the best chance of good cosmetic outcome.

5 ROSACEA – EPIDEMIOLOGY AND PATHOPHYSIOLOGY

INTRODUCTION

ROSACEA is a common cutaneous disorder that may present with a variety of clinical manifestations, including ocular involvement. It is, however, precisely because of such variability in presentation that a set of specific diagnostic criteria has long been elusive. Such pervasive confusion complicates not only clinical diagnosis and eventual choice of treatment modalities, but also research studies and investigations into the pathophysiology of this disease. A relatively recent consensus by a panel of experts established a new classification system based on relatively specific clinical features (Wilkin *et al.* 2002). Though not without its shortcomings, such a system represents an extremely important advance in rosacea.

EPIDEMIOLOGY

Although diagnosed in patients of most ethnicities and races (**51, 52**), rosacea is most prevalent in fair-skinned individuals, especially of Northern and Eastern European descent, and is estimated to occur in 2.1–10% in this population (Bamford *et al.* 2006; Berg & Liden 1989). Unfortunately, large epidemiological studies have been hampered by the above-mentioned lack of precise and uniform clinical criteria that define this disease.

Only a handful of studies have carefully examined the prevalence of rosacea by gender and age. In a frequently-cited study of Swedish office employees, rosacea was found to be nearly three times more common in women than in men (Berg & Liden 1989). However, because of the selected study population, elderly patients were

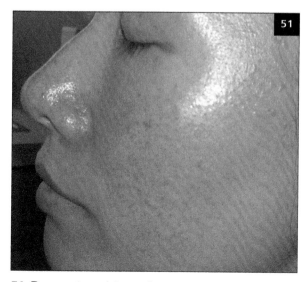

51 Rosacea in an Asian patient.

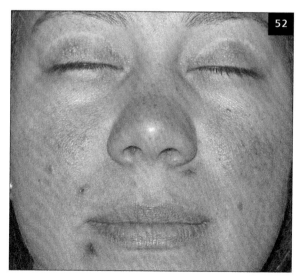

52 Rosacea in an Hispanic patient.

under-represented. Other studies have noted an overall equal prevalence in both genders, with a tendency toward earlier presentation in females compared to males (Kyriakis *et al.* 2005). Gender predisposition also depends on the individual rosacea subtype, with rhynophyma occurring predominantly in male patients (Kyriakis *et al.* 2005).

Overall, rosacea is most frequently diagnosed in patients between the ages of 30 and 50 years; however, presentation in the seventh, eighth, and even in the ninth decade in not unusual (Kyriakis *et al.* 2005). Childhood rosacea cases, though rare, have been documented in the literature (Chamaillard *et al.* 2008; Drolet & Paller 1992; Erzurum *et al.* 1993).

DEFINITION OF ROSACEA

No specific laboratory tests are available for rosacea; thus, a system of signs and symptoms must be utilized to define this disease. As per the expert committee consensus, rosacea may be diagnosed when one or more of the primary features are present, most commonly on the convex surfaces of the central face. The primary features include flushing (or transient erythema), persistent erythema, papules and pustules, and telangiectasias (Wilkin *et al.* 2002). Additional secondary features may include burning or stinging, rough and scaly appearance likely as a result of local irritation, edema, elevated red plaques, peripheral localization, ocular manifestations, and phymatous changes. Other authors have, however, suggested that these criteria may not be specific enough. They have thus proposed that persistent centrofacial erythema lasting at least 3 months with a tendency toward periocular sparing is most characteristic of rosacea (Crawford *et al.* 2004).

Awareness of the potential rosacea mimickers is important. These include erythema and telangiectasias frequently noted in lupus erythematosus, dermatomyositis, and other connective tissue diseases, flushing associated with the carcinoid syndrome and mastocytosis, and plethora seen in polycythemia vera. Finally, if suspected, allergic contact dermatitis and photosensitivity can be excluded with the help of patch testing and phototesting, respectively.

ROSACEA SUBTYPES

Once diagnosed, each case of rosacea should be further classified as one of four recognized subtypes (*Table 6*).

Erythematotelangiectatic subtype
Papulopustular subtype
Phymatous subtype
Ocular subtype
Granulomatous variant*
*currently not recognized as a separate subtype

Table 6 Rosacea classification

This is an essential part of the diagnosis, as it has a direct impact on the choice of treatment modalities and the prognosis. The subtype is determined based on the predominant features present in a given patient. According to the expert committee, rosacea may be subdivided into erythematotelangiectatic (ET), papulopustular (PP), phymatous, and ocular subtypes, with granulomatous rosacea considered a special variant of the disease (Wilkin *et al.* 2002). On the other hand, several conditions previously considered variants of rosacea have now been reclassified as separate diagnostic entities. These include rosacea fulminans, also known as pyoderma faciale, steroid-induced acneiform eruption, and perioral dermatitis. It should, however, be noted that some authors consider rosacea to be a much more polymorphic disease with many more subtypes than those recognized by the expert panel (Kligman 2006). Still, the following discussion will focus on the latter, more widely-accepted classification system.

Erythematotelangiectatic subtype

Patients who belong to this subtype typically present with persistent centrofacial erythema and an extensive history of prolonged flushing in response to various stimuli (**53, 54**). Although not required for the diagnosis of this subtype, facial telangiectasias may also be present in the affected areas (**55**). Flushing may affect not only the central portions of the face, but also the ears, neck, and chest (Marks & Jones 1969). Unlike physiologic flushing, or blushing, prolonged facial vasodilation (lasting 10 minutes or longer and often accompanied by burning or stinging) is typically observed in such patients. It is important to note,

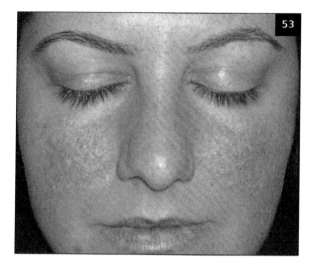

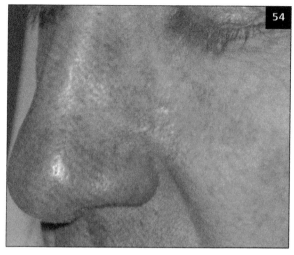

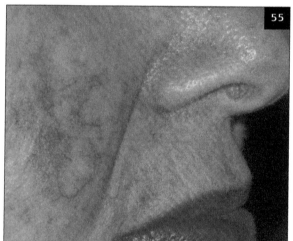

53 **Erythematotelangiectatic subtype** of rosacea.

54 **Erythematotelangiectatic subtype** of rosacea resembling the stigmata of alcoholism.

55 **Extensive telangiectasias** in erythematotelangiectatic rosacea.

however, that flushing associated with rosacea is never accompanied by sweating or light-headedness; in such cases, systemic causes of flushing should be sought. As well, perimenopausal flushing should not automatically evoke the diagnosis of rosacea, unless other symptoms and signs are present in a given patient.

The stimuli of flushing, also known as triggers, may vary among patients and most commonly include hot showers, the extremes of ambient temperatures, hot liquids, spicy foods, alcohol, exercise, and emotional stress (Greaves & Burova 1997; Higgins & du Vivier 1999; Wilkin 1981). In addition, various foods, such as citrus fruits and tomatoes, have been described as occasional triggers, and detailed food diaries may be helpful in some patients.

Patients with ET rosacea tend to exhibit poor tolerability of topically-applied products, often including those meant to ameliorate the condition. Itching, burning, and stinging following topical application are common complaints; over time, roughness and scaling may develop, likely as a consequence of low-grade irritation (Dahl 2001; Lonne-Rahm *et al.* 1999). Although patch testing may at times be useful in these patients, most cases of contact dermatitis associated with ET rosacea appear to be irritant, rather than allergic, in nature (Jappe *et al.* 2005).

Papulopustular subtype

This subtype of rosacea most resembles acne vulgaris, but lacks comedones. Patients present with persistent central facial erythema and transient papules and pustules, typically sparing the periocular regions (**56**). Edema may at times be present, but solid facial edema is rare (Harvey *et al.* 1998; Scerri & Saihan 1995). Flushing may occur, but is usually less common and less pronounced than that seen in patients with ET rosacea. Burning and stinging, as well as sensitivity to topical products, may be reported, but are also less frequent in PP rosacea as compared to the ET subtype (Lonne-Rahm *et al.* 1999). Additionally, telangiectasias may be difficult to discern, as they are often obscured by the background of erythema. Progression to the phymatous subtype may occur in severe cases, but is most often limited to the male patients. The reasons for such a gender difference, however, are not fully understood.

Phymatous subtype

Phymatous rosacea is defined by thickened skin and irregular surface nodularities (Wilkin *et al.* 2002). Patulous follicles, as well as persistent erythema, papules and pustules, and telangiectasias, are also frequently seen in the areas of involvement. Although most common on the nose, where it is known as rhinophyma (**57**), this type of rosacea may also occur on the chin, forehead, ears, and eyelids. Despite a common misperception, most cases of rhinophyma are not associated with alcohol consumption (Curnier & Choudhary 2004). Four variants of rhinophyma, glandular, fibrous, fibroangiomatous, and actinic, have been recognized based on clinical and histological differences and a variety of grading scales have been devised (Aloi *et al.* 2000; Freeman 1970; Jansen & Plewig 1998). In severe cases, secondary nasal airway obstruction may occur; however, bony and cartilaginous structures are typically not affected (Rohrich *et al.* 2002).

Ocular subtype

Ocular rosacea should be considered in patients with such symptoms as burning, stinging, and itching of the eyes, foreign body sensation, light sensitivity, and blurred vision. Clinically, blepharitis and conjunctivitis are the most common presentations of ocular rosacea. Additional findings may include watery or dry eyes, interpalpebral conjunctival hyperemia, conjunctival telangiectasias, irregularity of the lid margin, eyelid and periocular erythema and edema, meibomian gland

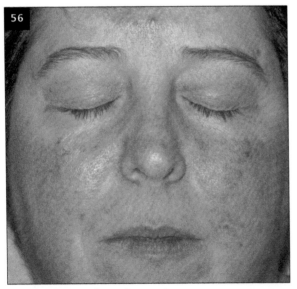

56 Papulopustular subtype of rosacea.

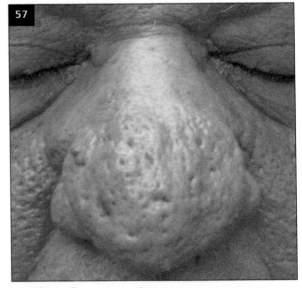

57 Rhinophyma in an African-American patient.

dysfunction, and recurrent chalazia (Akpek *et al.* 1997; Chen & Crosby 1997; Lemp *et al.* 1984) (**58**). Although infrequent, keratitis, episcleritis, corneal perforations, and iritis may also occur and are potentially serious complications that may lead to blindness or require enucleation (Akpek *et al.* 1997; Browning & Proia 1986).

The true incidence of ocular rosacea is difficult to ascertain secondary to conflicting reports in ophthalmologic and dermatologic literature, with estimates ranging from less than 5% to as high as 58% of all rosacea patients (Kligman 2006; Starr & Macdonald 1969). Ocular signs and symptoms may precede skin involvement in up to 20% of patients; however, the diagnosis of ocular rosacea without cutaneous findings is difficult, as most manifestations are nonspecific (Browning & Proia 1986).

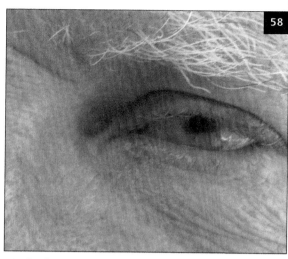

58 Ocular rosacea.

Granulomatous variant

Classified by the expert panel as a special variant of rosacea, granulomatous rosacea often lacks many of the characteristic findings of the classic disease, including persistent erythema, flushing, and telangiectasias. It is also likely that lupus miliaris disseminatus faciei and granulomatous rosacea represent the same disorder, although this view is controversial (van de Scheur *et al.* 2003). Clinically, individual firm 1–5 mm brown-red to yellow papules and nodules appear on relatively normal, noninflamed skin. Involvement is not limited to the convexities of the face, with the eyelids, cheeks, and the upper lip being the most commonly-affected locations. Without treatment, lesions eventually resolve with scarring. Histologically, epithelioid granulomas with or without caseation necrosis have been observed; however, there is no relationship to *Mycobacterium tuberculosis* infection (Helm *et al.* 1991). Some authors believe that because of the significant clinical and histological differences from the other subtypes of rosacea, the granulomatous variant may, in fact, represent a distinct diagnostic entity (Crawford *et al.* 2004).

PATHOPHYSIOLOGY OF ROSACEA

The study into the pathophysiology of rosacea has long been hampered by the lack of specific diagnostic criteria. In addition, many studies fail to specify the breakdown of the various subtypes, which may potentially have varied pathogenic mechanisms. Nonetheless, several fundamental findings have recently been made, and our understanding of the pathophysiological factors underlying the development of rosacea will likely improve significantly in the near future. Numerous mechanisms have been proposed over the years, including vascular abnormalities, inflammation and dermal matrix degradation, climactic exposures, pilosebaceous unit abnormalities, and various microbial organisms, and will now be examined at length.

Vascular abnormalities

Since flushing is often exaggerated in rosacea patients, inherent vascular abnormalities have been proposed as a causative factor in the pathogenesis of this disorder (Wilkin 1994). In a small study, a normal physiological response to hyperthermia of shunting blood away from facial circulation in order to increase blood flow to the brain was absent in rosacea patients (Brinnel *et al.* 1989). Rosacea patients have also been shown to flush more easily in response to various thermal stimuli. In the case of oral exposure to heat, such as that seen with ingestion of hot liquids, a countercurrent heat exchange between the internal jugular vein and the common carotid artery may be produced, thus triggering an anterior hypothalamic thermoregulatory reflex, resulting in cutaneous vasodilation (Wilkin 1981).

Why is flushing localized to the face? Both vasodilation in general and flushing in particular are controlled by neural stimuli and humoral factors. In fact, it has been shown that the proportional vasodilatory response to both neurally- and humorally-mediated triggers is the same in cutaneous vasculature of the face and of the forearm (Wilkin 1988). However, the baseline cutaneous blood flow has been shown to be higher and the blood vessels larger, more numerous, and closer to the surface on the face as compared to other parts of the body (Tur et al. 1983; Wilkin 1988). Of interest, since both the blood flow and pain perception are regulated by C nerve fibers, low heat pain threshold has been found in the affected areas in patients with PP rosacea (Guzman-Sanchez et al. 2007).

More recently, the role of angiogenesis and vascular factors has been investigated. An increased expression of vascular endothelial growth factor (VEGF) and vascular endothelial marker CD31 has been demonstrated in the affected skin of rosacea patients (Gomaa et al. 2007). VEGF plays a dual role by inducing angiogenesis and by increasing vascular permeability with subsequent leakage of various proinflammatory factors, which may further contribute to the pathogenesis of the disease. In addition, tetracycline and similar agents work, at least in part, by inhibiting angiogenesis, further suggesting the role of neovascularization in rosacea (Dan et al. 2008; Fife et al. 2000; Gilbertson-Beadling et al. 1995). Of note, a high expression of D2-40, a marker of lymphatic vessels, in the affected skin has been demonstrated in both early and long-standing disorder, suggesting lymphangiogenesis as an early pathological process in rosacea (Gomaa et al. 2007).

Inflammation and dermal matrix degradation

Abnormalities of dermal connective tissue as seen in rosacea patients may be caused by the preceding vascular derangements (Neumann & Frithz 1998). Thus, inherent or acquired vasculopathy and the increased expression of VEGF may lead to leaky blood vessels and dermal accumulation of cytokines and other inflammatory mediators with subsequent dermal matrix deterioration.

On the other hand, some researchers suggest a primary role for inflammation and connective tissue

damage in the pathogenesis of vascular changes associated with the disease (Bevins & Liu 2007; Millikan 2004; Yamasaki et al. 2007). This is supported, in part, by the finding that ectatic blood vessels in rosacea are still able to dilate and contract in response to vasoactive agents (Borrie 1955a, b). Instead, solar exposure, as will be discussed in the next section, may cause deterioration of collagen and elastic fibers, resulting in poor structural support for the cutaneous vasculature (Fisher et al. 1999).

The weakened or leaky blood vessel walls may lead to the extravasation of proinflammatory mediators and neutrophil chemotaxis. Activated neutrophils release reactive oxygen species (ROS) and various matrix metalloproteinases (MMPs), which further contribute to dermal matrix degradation and perpetuate the inflammatory response (Akamatsu et al. 1990; Jones 2004). Moreover, a decrease in the capacity of the antioxidant defense system, including superoxide dismutase, has been demonstrated in severe rosacea (Oztas et al. 2003). In addition, a study by Yazici et al. (2006) showed a significant correlation between rosacea and specific genetic polymorphisms in the glutathione S-transferase genes, also responsible for cellular defense against ROS damage. The newest findings involving the action of cathelicidin in the pathophysiology of rosacea gives further credence to the primary role of the immune system in rosacea (Yamasaki et al. 2007). These important findings will be discussed in a later section.

Climactic exposures

The notion that climactic exposures, most notably solar radiation, may lead to the development of rosacea has been advocated by many investigators (Wilkin 1994). This is supported by the observation that convex, sun-exposed surfaces are typically involved, sparing the sun-protected periorbital and submental areas. Prolonged ultraviolet (UV) radiation leads to the degradation of the elastic fiber network and collagen fibers in the dermis, resulting in the accumulation of solar elastotic material. As previously discussed, this leads to a weakened support structure for cutaneous vasculature. In addition, an upregulation of VEGF and subsequent angiogenesis has been demonstrated following irradiation of skin with UV-B light (Yano et al. 2005).

On the other hand, if excessive sun exposure were the primary etiological factor for rosacea, significant actinic damage prior to the development of the disease, as evidenced by a high incidence of actinic keratoses, would be expected. However, a very large study documented an increase in actinic keratoses only in female rosacea patients, but not in male patients (Engel *et al.* 1988). Additionally, despite a common misperception, rosacea patients do not show increased photosensitivity compared to the normal population. In fact, minimum erythema dose of either UV-A or UV-B radiation in rosacea patients is not decreased (Lee & Koo 2005). Thus, flares in response to sun exposure may actually be a reaction to heat rather than the light itself (Kligman 2006).

Pilosebaceous unit abnormalities

Despite certain similarities to acne vulgaris, it is not entirely clear whether the inflammatory lesions of rosacea are follicle-based. One study showed that only 20% of papules had follicular origin, while most histological studies of ET and PP rosacea have documented a low rate of periadnexal inflammation (Marks & Harcourt-Webster 1969; Ramelet & Perroulaz 1988). On the other hand, the glandular type of rhinophyma has been shown to be folliculocentric (Aloi *et al.* 2000). As well, *Demodex folliculorum*, a follicle-based mite, has been investigated on multiple occasions for its possible etiological function in rosacea, as will be described below. Thus, additional, more rigorous histological studies may be necessary to determine the role of the pilosebaceous unit in the development of this disease.

Microbial organisms

Three microbial organisms have been proposed as potentially pathogenic in rosacea: *Demodex folliculorum*, *Bacillus oleronius*, and *Helicobacter pylori*.

Demodex mite is a common inhabitant of the human skin. In fact, a prevalence of nearly 100% has been demonstrated in healthy adult subjects using the modern, more sensitive identification techniques (Crosti *et al.* 1983). Mite density in tissue samples tends to increase with age, paralleling a similar trend in rosacea incidence (Andrews 1982). As its full name implies, *Demodex* usually resides in the follicles, most commonly on the nose, forehead, and cheeks

(Bonnar *et al.* 1993). It has been suggested that an extrafollicular localization in the dermis may be pathogenic, as it then leads to a pronounced inflammatory reaction (Ecker & Winkelmann 1979; Hoekzema *et al.* 1995).

Numerous studies have attempted to compare mite density in rosacea versus healthy patients. In two studies that employed highly sensitive techniques, the density of *Demodex* was found to be significantly higher in PP rosacea patients as compared to age-matched controls, whereas no statistical difference was demonstrated for patients with the ET subtype (Erbagci & Ozgoztasi 1998; Forton & Seys 1993). It is unclear, however, whether this difference in mite population is pathogenic or, instead, reflective of the presence of abnormal antimicrobial peptides, as will be discussed in the next section (Bevins & Liu 2007). Of interest, the *Demodex* density does not seem to decrease when standard oral antibiotics are used for the treatment of rosacea (Bonnar *et al.* 1993). In addition, though some investigators have noted perifollicular inflammatory infiltrates in the presence of the *Demodex* mite (Forton 1986), others have noted a lack of such correlation (Marks & Harcourt-Webster 1969; Ramelet & Perroulaz 1988). These discrepancies may, however, be secondary to the difficulty in detecting mites on standard histological sections.

More recently, a potential role of a bacterial agent found inside the *Demodex* mites, *Bacillus oleronius*, has been investigated. When isolated, this bacterium was able to stimulate an immune response and caused peripheral mononuclear cell proliferation in 73% of patients with PP rosacea as compared to 29% of the control population (Lacey *et al.* 2007). Further studies are necessary; however, if these findings are confirmed, *D. folliculorum* may turn out to be essential as a vector of a pathogenic agent.

Multiple studies have concentrated on the potential role of *Helicobacter pylori* in the etiology of rosacea; however, currently available data do not support such a role. Although extremely common in the general population, *H. pylori* rarely causes symptoms. Nonetheless, most cases of peptic ulcer disease and gastritis have now been linked to this organism, and some correlations between these gastrointestinal conditions and rosacea, such as seasonal variability, have been proposed.

A high prevalence of *H. pylori* in rosacea patients has been noted in several studies (Rebora *et al.* 1995; Szlachcic *et al.* 1999); most others have refuted such findings when the prevalence is compared to a control population (Jones *et al.* 1998; Sharma *et al.* 1998; Utas *et al.* 1999). Likewise, eradication of the bacterium did or did not improve the symptoms and signs of rosacea, depending on the study (Bamford *et al.* 1999; Gedik *et al.* 2005; Herr & You 2000; Utas *et al.* 1999). It should, however, be noted that the medications typically used to eradicate *H. pylori*–in particular, metronidazole–are known for their beneficial effect in rosacea, and the effectiveness of therapy does not, therefore, establish a causal association. In one study, elevated plasma levels of tumor necrosis factor (TNF)-alpha and interleukin (IL)-8 in response to *H. pylori* were demonstrated in patients with symptoms of gastritis. Following treatment, most patients with concurrent rosacea experienced a significant improvement in their cutaneous condition, while their plasma cytokine levels normalized (Szlachcic *et al.* 1999). However, significantly elevated gastrin levels were also noted prior to therapy and may have been responsible for variations in skin temperature and vasomotor instability. In summary, without additional rigorous, well-controlled prospective studies a role for *H. pylori* in the pathogenesis of rosacea is doubtful.

Newest findings

The latest findings in the pathophysiology of rosacea seem to link many of the above-mentioned etiological factors; nonetheless, certain questions remain unanswered at this time. In a recent study, an overexpression and abnormal processing of cathelicidin have been demonstrated (Yamasaki *et al.* 2007). Also known as anti-microbial peptides for their action against Gram-positive and Gram-negative bacteria and some viruses, cathelicidins are part of the innate immune system with important links to adaptive immunity (Di Nardo *et al.* 2008; Howell *et al.* 2004; Nizet *et al.* 2001; Rosenberger *et al.* 2004; Yang *et al.* 2000). In the skin, cathelicidin is first secreted as a proprotein, known as 18-kDa cationic antimicrobial protein (CAP18), which is then cleaved by a serine protease, known as stratum corneum tryptic enzyme (SCTE) or kallikrein 5, to the active peptides (Yamasaki *et al.* 2006).

Facial skin affected by rosacea demonstrated a highly-elevated expression of SCTE in all layers of the epidermis compared to normal facial skin, where the expression was also limited to the superficial layers. This was accompanied by a significantly higher expression of a biologically-active cathelicidin fragment, LL-37, and by the expression of several other fragments not encountered in normal skin. Furthermore, injection of these molecules into healthy mice rapidly induced clinical findings of erythema and vascular dilatation, as well as cutaneous inflammation, in a dose-dependent manner. Additionally, injection of SCTE into mice also resulted in similar changes. Finally, protease activity was also shown to be higher in facial skin as compared to other parts of the body, corresponding to the typical localization of rosacea (Yamasaki *et al.* 2007).

Elevated levels of LL-37 lead to an increase in IL-8, a neutrophil chemoattractive cytokine (Yamasaki *et al.* 2007; Yang *et al.* 2000). As previously described, the influx of neutrophils initiates an inflammatory cascade and tissue degradation through the release of ROS and MMPs. Additionally, LL-37 is a strong angiogenic agent, thus further contributing to the observed rosacea phenotype (Koczulla *et al.* 2003).

Nonetheless, several questions persist: First, a complete characterization of the additional proteases and protease inhibitors involved in the homeostasis of LL-37 is critical. Second, although the above findings represent a major breakthrough in the pathophysiology of rosacea, the initial insult or defect that eventuates in the overexpression of SCTE and cathelicidin LL-37 still needs to be identified. Finally, future research studies may attempt to develop specific mechanism-based treatments afforded by these new findings.

6 ROSACEA – CURRENT MEDICAL THERAPEUTICS

INTRODUCTION

As with acne vulgaris, multiple topical and oral agents have been tried over the years for the treatment of rosacea. In fact, a large portion of the medications introduced in Chapter 2 of this book have been successfully utilized in rosacea (Table 7). These are especially important in the treatment of the acne–rosacea overlap, where clinical components of both diseases coexist in the same patient. On the other hand, additional therapeutic agents that may improve one disorder may not be useful in or even aggravate the other disease (Tables 8, 9). Rather than repeat the information already contained in a prior chapter, this chapter will focus mainly on the medications found to be of exclusive value in the treatment of rosacea and will only briefly touch on the previously-covered, but otherwise useful, rosacea agents. For the latter group of medications, the reader is invited to revisit the appropriate sections of Chapter 2. In addition, wherever available, current information on the proposed mechanism of action of the therapeutic agents will also be presented.

Although efficacious in the treatment of papulopustular (PP) rosacea, both oral and topical agents tend to have less of an impact on the erythema of erythematotelangiectatic (ET) rosacea, and even so on telangiectasias. On the other hand, vascular-specific lasers may be especially useful in such presentations and will be covered in Chapter 7.

GENERAL CONSIDERATIONS

Before the forthcoming discussion on topical and oral therapeutics in rosacea, some important general considerations will now be addressed. First, patient exposure to rosacea triggers, as presented in the previous chapter, must be minimized. Thus, patients should be educated on the avoidance of their specific flushing stimuli. Additionally, the National Rosacea

Agent	Mode
Clindamycin	Topical
Retinoids	Topical
Azelaic acid	Topical
Sulfur	Topical
Sodium sulfacetamide	Topical
Tetracyclines	Oral
Azithromycin	Oral
Isotretinoin	Oral

Table 7 Agents generally appropriate for the treatment of both rosacea and acne vulgaris

Agent	Mode
Metronidazole	Topical and oral
Tacrolimus	Topical
Pimecrolimus	Topical

Table 8 Agents generally appropriate for the treatment of rosacea, but not acne vulgaris

Agent	Mode
Benzoyl peroxide	Topical
Salicylic acid	Topical
Trimethoprim–sulfamethoxazole	Oral

Table 9 Agents generally appropriate for the treatment of acne vulgaris, but not rosacea

Society, which can be found on the internet at http://www.rosacea.org, is an excellent educational resource for the patients.

General skin care should be addressed early on in the treatment of the disease. As mentioned in the previous chapter, poor tolerability of topical products is commonly encountered in rosacea, especially the ET subtype. The resultant irritant dermatitis typically presents as roughness and scaling, sometimes accompanied by itching, burning, or stinging (Dahl 2001; Lonne-Rahm et al. 1999). Thus, the selection of nonirritating cleansers, moisturizers, and make-up is essential, as harsh daily skin care regimens may negatively affect skin barrier function (Del Rosso 2005; Draelos 2004, 2006a; Laquieze et al. 2007). Some patients may also benefit from the use of green-tinted moisturizers and other green-colored cosmetics, as these tend to camouflage excessive facial redness. A tan-colored foundation can then be applied to match the patient's desired skin tone (Draelos 2008). Finally, photoprotection is advocated by many practitioners; however, the exact role of ultraviolet radiation in the pathogenesis of rosacea is still debated (Engel et al. 1988; Kligman 2006; Lee & Koo 2005, Wilkin 1994). When utilized, sun blocks containing zinc oxide or titanium dioxide tend to be well-tolerated by rosacea patients.

TOPICAL AGENTS

As with acne vulgaris, topical agents may be used alone or in combination with oral agents for maximum effect, especially during acute flares of the disease. In addition, topical therapy is generally required for long-term maintenance of remission (Dahl et al. 1998; Nielsen 1983). As mentioned above, rosacea patients may experience significant skin irritability, occasionally necessitating a discontinuation of the very same medications typically prescribed to improve the condition. This distinctive feature of the disease should be considered whenever a flare is observed with a new topical agent, especially if accompanied by itching, burning, or stinging.

Antibiotics

Metronidazole is one of the most commonly used topical agents in the treatment of rosacea. Although infrequently used in this condition, the oral form is also available for the more severe or recalcitrant cases. Topical metronidazole is available in different countries in a gel, cream, and lotion formulations, with concentrations ranging from 0.75 to 1%. Formulations may be used daily to twice daily (Yoo et al. 2006). A combination of topical metronidazole cream and sunscreen is also available outside the US. Oral metronidazole is available in 200 mg, 250 mg, 400 mg, and 500 mg tablets, as well as 750 mg extended-release tablets. The original study by Pye & Burton (1976) utilized a 200 mg dose taken twice daily, while later studies used a total of 500 mg per day (Aizawa et al. 1992).

Metronidazole is a synthetic nitroimidazole antibiotic. It is active against a variety of Gram-positive and Gram-negative, as well as some anerobic, bacteria and certain protozoans, likely through the disruption of microbial DNA (Lamp et al.1999). However, its role in the treatment of rosacea appears to involve a different mechanism of action, as bacteria are unlikely to be involved in the pathophysiology of the condition. Thus, it has been demonstrated that metronidazole possesses significant anti-inflammatory properties in the skin. Specifically, the agent was found to modulate neutrophil function by suppressing neutrophil-generated reactive oxygen species (ROS) in a dose-related manner (Akamatsu et al. 1990; Miyachi et al. 1986). More recently, inherent ROS scavenging and inactivating properties of metronidazole were also demonstrated in a skin lipid model (Narayanan et al. 2007).

Systemic absorption following cutaneous application appears to be very low (Elewski 2007). On the other hand, oral bioavailability of metronidazole is very high at over 90%. It is widely distributed following oral administration, including into breast milk and across the placenta. Studies on such distribution following cutaneous application to intact skin are lacking.

Adverse effects following topical application to skin are few and typically include symptoms of localized irritant dermatitis. Rare cases of allergic contact dermatitis (sometimes to the base rather than to metronidazole itself) have also been documented (Choudry et al. 2002; Madsen et al. 2007).

On the other hand, adverse effects associated with oral administration of metronidazole are fairly numerous and potentially serious, but are more frequent at higher doses and with long-term therapy (Martinez & Caumes 2001). These may include seizures, peripheral neuropathy, nausea, metallic taste, headaches, and various hypersensitivity reactions. In addition, oral metronidazole potentiates the anticoagulant effect of warfarin. However, the previously-accepted notion of a disulfiram-like reaction when the agent is co-administered with alcohol has recently been challenged (Visapaa et al. 2002; Williams & Woodcock 2000). Finally, it has been suggested that oral metronidazole and its metabolites may be mutagenic, though evidence from human studies is insufficient at this time (Bendesky et al. 2002; Menendez et al. 2002). Metronidazole in both topical and oral forms is an FDA pregnancy category B agent. It is excreted in breast milk following oral, but not topical, administration.

Topical clindamycin may also used in the treatment of inflammatory papules and pustules associated with rosacea. It is available in numerous formulations containing 1% clindamycin phosphate, including solutions, lotions, gels, and foams. In the treatment of rosacea, the gel preparation is usually tolerated better and is typically administered once to twice daily (Wilkin & DeWitt 1993). Clindamycin belongs to lincosamide family of antibacterial agents, though its mechanism of action in rosacea has not been studied directly. Recently, however, an in-vitro study demonstrated a direct scavenging effect of clindamycin phosphate on hydroxyl radicals, suggesting a potential antioxidant action in rosacea (Sato et al. 2007). The systemic absorption, pharmacology, and adverse effects of clindamycin have been covered extensively in a prior chapter. Topical clindamycin is an FDA pregnancy category B agent. The topical agent appears to be safe in lactating women, as no adverse effects have been documented in the infants of such patients.

Azelaic acid

Azelaic acid is a 9-carbon-chain dicarboxylic acid derived from Pityrosporum ovale. It is available as a 20% cream and, more recently, as a 15% gel. Although both formulations have been successfully used in the treatment of inflammatory rosacea (Bjerke et al. 1999; Elewski et al. 2003; Maddin 1999; Thiboutot et al. 2003), the cream preparation contains significantly larger amounts of emulsifiers, which may lead to a greater potential for skin irritation (Draelos 2006b). Additionally, the amount of the active ingredient delivered to the skin has been found to be significantly greater using the gel formulation than using the cream

(Maru et al. 1982). While the traditional rosacea regimen called for twice daily application of azelaic acid, the efficacy of once-daily administration has also been documented and may be associated with greater patient tolerability and dosing flexibility (Thiboutot et al. 2008).

The mechanism of action of azelaic acid in the treatment of rosacea has not been completely elucidated. As mentioned in Chapter 2, the agent has antiproliferative, antibacterial, and antikeratinizing properties; however, these actions are unlikely to account for the improvement noted in rosacea. Instead, similar to metronidazole, azelaic acid appears to be a potent inhibitor of neutrophil-generated ROS and to possess free-radical scavenging properties (Akamatsu et al. 1991; Passi et al. 1991a, b).

Although only local application-site adverse effects have been reported with topical azelaic acid, these appear to be somewhat more frequent than with topical metronidazole (Ziel et al. 2005). Pruritus, stinging, burning, erythema, and peeling are encountered most commonly. Azelaic acid is an FDA pregnancy category B agent. Since azelaic acid is normally present in most diets from its natural occurrence in cereals and other products, topical application of the agent is likely safe during lactation.

Sodium sulfacetamide and sulfur

These agents were introduced in Chapter 2 as effective therapeutic agents in the treatment of acne vulgaris. Likewise, both sodium sulfacetamide and sulfur have a long history of use in inflammatory rosacea (Lebwohl et al. 1995; Torok et al. 2005). Their mechanism of action in this condition is, however, unclear, but may involve anti-inflammatory properties of both agents.

The combination of the two agents is available outside of the U.K. in a number of creams, lotions, gels, suspensions, cleansers, and masks. The concentrations of these ingredients may vary, though a combination of 10% sodium sulfacetamide and 5% sulfur is encountered most commonly. These products are now experiencing resurgence due to the recent availability of odor-masking formulations. Once- to twice-daily application regimen is most commonly used in the treatment of rosacea.

Adverse effects following topical application of sodium sulfacetamide/sulfur combination products are generally mild and limited to localized irritant dermatitis with erythema, itching, burning, itching, and scaling.

The incidence of such reactions appears to be somewhat higher compared to those from topical metronidazole (Torok *et al.* 2005). Although sulfur does not cross-react with sulfonamides, sodium sulfacetamide does, making the combination contraindicated in patients with allergic reactions to 'sulfa' drugs. Both topical sulfur and sodium sulfacetamide are FDA pregnancy category C agents. Although the excretion in breast milk has not been studied with either, an increased risk of kernicterus in nursing infants has been documented with oral administration of sulfonamides.

Retinoids

As introduced in Chapter 2, retinoids are used extensively in the treatment of acne vulgaris. Though their use in rosacea is significantly less common, it has been evaluated in several studies (Altinyazar *et al.* 2005; Ertl *et al.* 1994).

The mechanism of action of retinoids in rosacea is not completely clear. Various anti-inflammatory properties of retinoids, including an antioxidant effect on the neutrophil system, have been demonstrated (Liu *et al.* 2005; Tenaud *et al.* 2007; Yoshioka *et al.* 1986). It has also been suggested that an additional mechanism may involve down-regulation of angiogenesis associated with the disease. To that effect, it has been shown that retinoids have an inhibitory effect on the expression of vascular endothelial growth factor (VEGF) and its receptor, though this effect is not mediated by the retinoic acid receptors (RARS) (Cho *et al.* 2005; Lachgar *et al.* 1999). Future studies will need to determine whether additional anti-inflammatory or antiproliferative properties of retinoids may be involved in the improvement of symptoms and signs of rosacea.

Although multiple formulations of retinoids are currently on the market, tazarotene is rarely used in rosacea due to its somewhat higher potential for local irritation. Other topical retinoids currently available in different formulations in different countries include tretinoin and adapalene. Tretinoin is available in cream, solution (with erythromycin outside the US), and gel forms, with concentrations ranging from 0.01% to 0.1%. Slightly less-irritating microsphere and delayed-release gel preparations are also available in some countries. Adapalene is available as a 0.1% cream, solution, and gel, as well as a 0.3% gel. Retinoids are typically used once daily, most commonly at night. This is especially important for tretinoin, which is photolabile (Shroot 1998).

Adverse effects associated with the use of topical retinoids in the treatment of rosacea are generally limited to localized irritation. This typically manifests as erythema and scaling, as well as pruritus, burning, or stinging. Adapalene may be associated with a slightly reduced risk of these side-effects, as is tretinoin incorporated into microspheres or into a polyolprepolymer-2 gel (Berger *et al.* 2007; Skov *et al.* 1997). Both topical tretinoin and adapalene are FDA pregnancy category C agents. Though not extensively studied, their use during lactation is inadvisable.

ORAL AGENTS

Oral agents are frequently utilized as part of a multiagent regimen in the setting of acute rosacea flares (**59, 60**). Once the flare has resolved, the oral agent may be discontinued, with remission maintained through the use of topical therapies, as described above.

Antibiotics

Among the oral agents used in the treatment of rosacea, the tetracycline family of antibiotics is employed most often. With rising concerns about the emergence of resistant bacterial strains, the recognition of anti-inflammatory properties of these agents with subsequent development of lower-dose regimens represents an important therapeutic advancement. The most commonly-used agents in this category include tetracycline (oxytetracycline and tetracycline hydrochloride), minocycline, and doxycycline. Tetracycline is available as 250 mg or 500 mg tablets or capsules, usually taken twice daily. Minocycline is formulated as capsules or tablets, with doses ranging from 50 to 100 mg twice daily. Finally, doxycycline is available in capsules, tablets, and enteric-coated tablets in 20, 50, 75, and 100 mg dosages typically administered twice daily. Additionally, a 40 mg once-daily formulation, containing 30 mg of immediate-release and 10 mg of delayed-release doxycycline, is now available and has been approved by the FDA for this condition.

As the name implies, tetracyclines feature a tetracyclic naphthacene carboxamide ring structure (Sapadin & Fleischmajer 2006). While their antibacterial activity has been appreciated for decades, the anti-inflammatory properties of these agents have

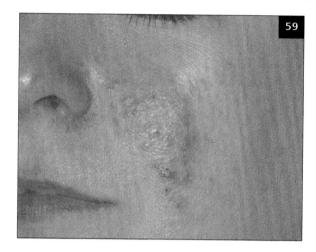

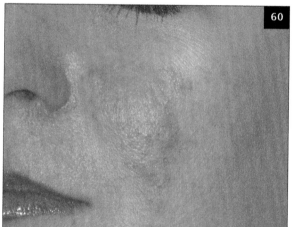

59, 60 Papulopustular rosacea. 59 During an acute flare. 60 Following 3 weeks of combination therapy using oral low-dose doxycycline and topical 1% metronidazole gel.

to upregulate anti-inflammatory cytokines, and to down-regulate proinflammatory cytokines (Akamatsu *et al.* 1992; Amin *et al.* 1996; Esterly *et al.* 1978, 1984; Golub *et al.* 1995; Kloppenburg *et al.* 1995; Sainte-Marie *et al.* 1999). Furthermore, both minocycline and doxycycline have been shown to inhibit VEGF-induced angiogenesis, which may, at least partially, be responsible for the formation of telangiectasias in rosacea (Guerin *et al.* 1992; Tamargo *et al.* 1991; Yao *et al.* 2004, 2007).

The pharmacokinetics, adverse effects, and drug interactions of the tetracycline family of antibiotics have been extensively covered in Chapter 2 of this book. The reader may wish to review the corresponding section of that chapter at this time. Tetracyclines have important adverse effects on the developing bones and teeth; thus, all are designated as FDA pregnancy category D agents. Tetracyclines are also excreted in breast milk and are, therefore, contraindicated in nursing mothers.

Azithromycin is a macrolide antibiotic with known antibacterial, as well as anti-inflammatory, properties. It has also been used for the treatment of rosacea, though, due in part to its long half-life, various regimens have been employed (Fernandez-Obregon 1994; Modi *et al.* 2008; Sehgal *et al.* 2008). Azithromycin is available as 250, 500, and 600 mg tablets, 250 mg and 500 mg capsules, as powder for oral suspension, and as an extended-release oral suspension.

Multiple anti-inflammatory properties of macrolides have been demonstrated and may account for the utility of azithromycin in rosacea. Thus, these agents have been shown to inhibit neutrophil migration and chemotaxis through the down-regulation of adhesion molecules and selectins and the up-regulation of interleukin (IL)-8 and leukotriene B4 production, and to inhibit proinflammatory cytokines (Ianaro *et al.* 2000; Labro 1998). Azithromycin has also been demonstrated to possess antioxidant properties through the modification of neutrophil oxidative metabolism and ROS production (Bakar *et al.* 2007; Kadota *et al.* 1998; Levert *et al.* 1998).

Though rare, gastrointestinal adverse effects, typically nausea and diarrhea, are most commonly encountered with azithromycin. Overall, azithromycin is tolerated significantly better than erythromycin, also a macrolide antibiotic. Azithromycin is an FDA pregnancy category B agent. It also appears to be safe during lactation.

only recently been recognized. In the process, tetracyclines have been shown to affect many of the inflammatory pathways thought to be involved in the pathogenesis of rosacea. Thus, these agents have been shown to inhibit neutrophil chemotaxis and neutrophil generation of ROS, to scavenge for free radicals, to inhibit matrix metalloproteinases (MMPs),

Isotretinoin

The use of isotretinoin, or 13-*cis* retinoic acid, in rosacea has been less extensive as compared to that in acne vulgaris. Nonetheless, this may be a valuable agent in severe and recalcitrant cases of the inflammatory (PP) subtype of the disease. In addition, its beneficial effect in rhinophyma and rosacea fulminans, extremely treatment-resistant presentations of rosacea, has also been demonstrated (Jansen *et al*. 1994; Jansen & Plewig 1998). Isotretinoin is available as 5, 10, 20, 30, and 40 mg capsules and is administered once daily with fatty meals to improve absorption.

As with acne vulgaris, numerous dosing regimens have been attempted in studies on treatment of rosacea. Originally, doses of 0.5–2 mg/kg/day have been evaluated and found to result in significant and long-term improvement in the inflammatory lesions of rosacea (Hoting *et al*. 1986; Schell *et al*. 1987; Turjanmaa & Reunala 1987). However, since the condition tends to be chronic and typically associated with remissions and relapses, long-term or continuous regimens have been advocated by some authors. However, in order to limit the cumulative dose of the agent, low-dose isotretinoin therapy (typically 10–20 mg daily, but at times as low as 20 mg weekly) has been proposed (Erdogan *et al*. 1998; Ertl *et al*. 1994; Hofer 2004). Such regimens tend to incur fewer adverse effects, though recurrences are common following discontinuation of therapy.

Although not completely elucidated, the mechanism of action of oral isotretinoin in rosacea may involve its numerous anti-inflammatory and antiproliferative properties. For example, isotretinoin has been demonstrated to inhibit neutrophil and monocyte chemotaxis, as well as neutrophil production of ROS (Camisa *et al*. 1982; Falcon *et al*. 1986; Norris *et al*. 1987; Orfanos & Bauer 1983). Furthermore, its antiproliferative effect on endothelial cells has also been demonstrated, resulting in decreased angiogenesis (Lee *et al*. 1992). Future studies will need to confirm the relative contribution of these or other effects to the clinical improvement associated with the use of this agent in rosacea.

Important pharmacokinetic data, an extensive review of the numerous potential adverse effects associated with oral isotretinoin, as well as several important drug interactions have been presented in Chapter 2 and should be revisited by the reader at this time. Oral isotretinoin is associated with severe teratogenicity and is, therefore, an FDA pregnancy category X agent. Its use in the US is regulated through a stringent online monitoring system. Oral isotretinoin is also absolutely contraindicated in nursing mothers.

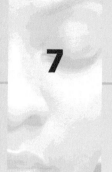

7 LASERS AND SIMILAR DEVICES IN THE TREATMENT OF ROSACEA

INTRODUCTION

Both topical and oral therapeutic agents introduced in the previous chapter have been shown to be of significant value in the treatment of rosacea. Clinical improvement, however, is usually most apparent in the inflammatory lesions associated with the disease, including papules and pustules, whereas the effect of these agents on erythema and especially telangiectasias tends to be limited at best. On the other hand, lasers and similar devices can predictably attain considerable amelioration in these latter lesions, thereby significantly improving the quality of life in rosacea patients, especially those with the erythematotelangiectatic subtype (Tan & Tope 2004).

This chapter will discuss established and time-honored light-based procedures currently used for the treatment of rosacea. Additionally, newer approaches currently being investigated for this condition will also be introduced.

GENERAL CONCEPTS AND MECHANISM OF ACTION

Although vascular lesions were effectively targeted by lasers since their introduction in medical science, early procedures were fraught with complications, such as scarring and dyschromia secondary to nonspecific coagulation necrosis of the superficial dermis. The treatments were finally revolutionized by the development of the theory of selective photothermolysis (Anderson & Parrish 1983). According to this theory, light beam can target a specific chromophore in the skin with minimal damage to surrounding structures through the selection of a proper wavelength, pulse duration, and fluence. In this manner, collateral damage to surrounding structures through the propagation of heat is minimized, also minimizing the risk of scarring and other long-term untoward events. Additional modifications to the theory,

as it applies to larger targets, such as blood vessels, were incorporated in the later expanded theory of selective photothermolysis (Altshuler et al. 2001).

The tissue chromophore in the treatment of erythema and telangiectasias of rosacea is oxyhemoglobin, which has major light absorption peaks at 418 nm, 542 nm, and 577 nm, with an additional broad absorption band from approximately 800 to 1100 nm (**61 overleaf**). It should be noted, however, that while the absorption of light by hemoglobin is highest at 418 nm, cutaneous penetration into the dermis by this short wavelength is insufficient to affect dermal vasculature. As the photons of lights are absorbed by the oxyhemoglobin molecule, electromagnetic energy is converted into heat. The heat then propagates to the red blood cells and, subsequently, to the blood vessel wall. Sufficient heating of the vessel wall results in coagulative damage to vascular lining, luminal closure, and eventual resorption of the vessel.

Thermal energy is confined to the target and injury to the surrounding dermis is minimized when the pulse duration of the laser beam, also known as the pulse width, is equal to or shorter than the thermal relaxation time (TRT) of the target. TRT is the time required for the target to cool to 1/e times the imparted energy, or by approximately 63%. TRT is directly proportional to the square of the target diameter. As a quick approximation, the TRT of a blood vessel, in seconds, may be estimated as a square of its diameter, in cm. Thus, a 1 mm (or 0.1 cm) telangiectasia has a TRT of approximately 10 ms (0.01 seconds). Pulse durations that are longer than the TRT of the target will lead to heat leakage from the target and potential damage to the surrounding tissues.

Another source of potential collateral damage during treatments is melanin, which also absorbs light within the visible and near-infrared portions of the electromagnetic spectrum. Thus, both the epidermal and the follicular melanin represent a potential

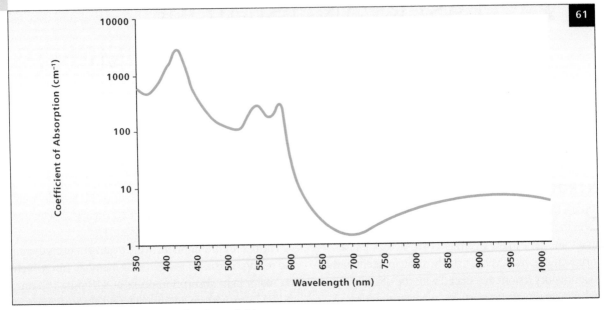

61 Light absorption spectrum of oxyhemoglobin.

competing chromophore when cutaneous erythema and telangiectasias are being treated with lasers and light-based devices. This is an important consideration in individuals with darker skin tones or those with facial hair. Thus, the various methods used to achieve greater target specificity in such cases will be covered with the individual systems.

Lasers and laser-like devices most commonly employed in the treatment of rosacea-associated erythema and telangiectasias include long-pulse pulsed-dye lasers (PDLs) and intense pulsed light (IPL) sources. In addition, a 532-nm potassium titanyl phosphate (KTP) laser and a 1064-nm neodymium:yttrium–aluminum–garnet (Nd:YAG) laser are also frequently utilized for this indication. These systems will now be examined in depth.

PREOPERATIVE CARE

Laser- and light-based treatment of rosacea is generally well-tolerated with relatively little preoperative preparation. Since makeup can both reflect and absorb various wavelengths of light, it is imperative that patients carefully remove all makeup and other facial products before the procedure. Most patients being treated for rosacea do not require topical anesthesia for pain control. As will be discussed below, epidermal cooling during the procedure helps to reduce patient discomfort. Additionally, topical anesthesia causes vasoconstriction, resulting in the loss of tissue chromophore. Nonetheless, a topical anesthetic cream, such as a mixture of topical 2.5% lidocaine and 2.5% prilocaine, or regional nerve blocks can be employed in exquisitely sensitive patients.

Finally, as mentioned above, melanin represents a competing chromophore when rosacea is being treated with lasers and light systems. This includes retinal melanin, thus obligating the practitioner to utilize wavelength-specific protective goggles both for the patient and the assisting staff.

PULSED-DYE LASERS

Pulsed dye laser (PDL) was the first laser to be designed in compliance with the theory of selective photothermolysis and was introduced in 1986. The original system emitted light with a wavelength of 577 nm, thus corresponding to one of the major oxyhemoglobin absorption peaks. Subsequently, the wavelength was increased to 585 nm and, later, to

595 nm in order to increase cutaneous penetration without a significant compromise to vascular selectivity. Both wavelengths are currently in use in the numerous systems available today (*Table 10*). Of importance, the longer (595 nm) wavelength is associated with relatively lower absorption by oxyhemoglobin as compared to the 585 nm wavelength, thus requiring an increase in fluence of 20–50% (Tan & Tope 2004). Most modern PDLs feature adjustable pulse durations of up to 40 ms, allowing for the treatment of erythema and variously-sized telangiectasias of rosacea. The introduction of longer pulse durations also permitted effective treatment of facial telangiectasias without purpura, as will be discussed below.

Since the first study on the use of PDL in rosacea in 1991, several additional studies have confirmed this laser's utility for this indication, with documented improvement in erythema of up to 50% and that in telangiectasias of up to 75% after one to three treatment sessions (Clark *et al.* 2002; Lowe *et al.* 1991; Tan *et al.* 2004). Additionally, a significant reduction in the incidence of flushing, as well as cutaneous sensitivity to lactic acid, have also been noted (Clark *et al.* 2002; Lonne-Rahm *et al.* 2004; Tan & Tope 2004). However, several adverse effects have been noted in these studies, most importantly purpura that occurs in all treated patients. Purpura may last from 5 to 10 days and may result in significant downtime for the patient. Additionally, hyperpigmentation and crusting occurred in a very large number of patients, while cases of atrophic scarring were rare (Clark *et al.* 2002; Tan *et al.* 2004).

Several advances have been made to improve the safety and tolerability of PDL treatments of rosacea. First, 'subpurpuric' doses (achieved with longer pulse durations of 6–10 ms and lower fluences) were introduced. These settings cause immediate, short-lived purpura due to intravascular coagulation, but no purpura persisting beyond several seconds, indicating the lack of rupture of the blood vessel wall. Pulses are typically delivered with a 50% overlap to prevent a honeycomb-like or reticulated appearance. Although subpurpuric doses are less effective as compared to traditional settings, vessel clearance may be improved with pulse stacking (Iyer & Fitzpatrick 2005; Rohrer *et al.* 2004). When using this technique, three to four stacked pulses are delivered over the same area. Thus,

significant improvement in rosacea symptoms and signs has been reported following a single treatment with subpurpuric settings (Jasim *et al.* 2004); however, in our practice we have found that a larger number of sessions–typically between two and six performed every 4–6 weeks–are necessary in most patients. It should also be noted that, in accordance with the theory of selective photothermolysis, longer pulse durations allow smaller vessels sufficient time to dissipate heat to the surrounding tissue and thus escape coagulation. Thus, the background erythema of rosacea, thought to be related to the presence of numerous small-caliber vessels, may require shorter pulse durations and, consequently, result in a higher incidence of purpura (Bernstein & Kligman 2008).

Second improvement on the traditional PDL was the introduction of epidermal cooling, usually delivered as cryogen spray or chilled air. Epidermal cooling serves three main purposes: (1) epidermal protection, resulting in a lower incidence of adverse effects, especially in darker skin tones; (2) safe delivery of higher fluences to target vessels; and (3) anesthetic effect during laser pulsing. As a result of these improvements, serious or long-term complications from PDL treatment of rosacea are now uncommon. Mild-to-moderate erythema and edema are noted most frequently, but typically resolve within several hours. A cool gel pack or packed ice may be used to shorten the duration of such sequelae. Isolated patches of purpura are possible even

Name	Manufacturer	Wavelength (nm)	Cooling
NLite	USA Photonics	585	None
Vbeam Perfecta	Candela	595	Cryogen
V-Star	Cynosure	595	Air
Cynergy	Cynosure	595/1064 (Nd:YAG)	Air

Table 10 Examples of commercially-available pulsed-dye lasers

at subpurpuric doses and patients should be forewarned accordingly.

The duration of improvement in rosacea symptoms and signs following PDL treatments has not been adequately studied and appears to vary significantly. In one study, worsening of residual erythema was reported to occur anywhere between 6 months and 52 months following laser treatment, depending on the original number of treatment sessions (Tan *et al.* 2004). The longevity of improvement likely also depends on the frequency of post-treatment exposure to rosacea triggers.

INTENSE PULSED LIGHT SOURCES

Initially greeted with skepticism due to the polychromatic and noncoherent nature of the emitted light, IPL sources have been found to be invaluable in the treatment of rosacea (**62, 63**). IPL sources vary in their spectral output, but generally emit light in the range of 400–1400 nm (*Table 11*). This permits deep penetration into the dermis, thus affecting deeper cutaneous vasculature. Additionally, these systems are equipped with large spot sizes, allowing for rapid and effective coverage of extensive treatment areas. Finally, most systems feature contact cooling with a chilled sapphire tip, providing epidermal protection and anesthesia.

Though each individual system's spectral output is proprietary, as a general rule, most energy is delivered by light with shorter wavelengths, with relatively little output beyond 1000 nm. Vascular selectivity can then be achieved with the use of optical cut-off filters, available on most modern systems. These filters block light output below a specified wavelength. Thus, a system can be easily adjusted for various clinical indications and skin types. Additionally, variable pulse duration allows the practitioner to adjust treatment settings based on the size of telangiectasias present in a given patient.

Multiple studies have documented safe and effective improvement in erythema, telangiectasias, and flushing associated with rosacea (Angermeier 1999; Kawana *et al.* 2007; Mark *et al.* 2003; Papageorgiou *et al.* 2008; Schroeter *et al.* 2005; Taub 2003). Although direct comparison of results is difficult largely due to significant variations between the individual IPL systems, important correlations and treatment pearls can, nonetheless, be derived from such studies.

Most patients with skin types I–III without tan can be safely treated using cut-off filters of 530 or 560 nm. In our practice, we have noted a significant incidence of localized purpura associated with the use of a 515 nm filter. Since melanin absorption decreases with increasing wavelengths, the use of a 590 nm or higher filter is preferred in patients with a tan or a preponderance of pigmented lesions, such as ephelides or lentigos. Individuals with darker skin tones should be treated with even higher-rated filters, such as 640 nm and above.

Several systems can be used in double- or triple-pulsed mode. This permits a separation of one long pulse into several shorter pulses with an adjustable delay between the pulses. Such inter-pulse delay allows for safer delivery of light energy in the setting of higher fluences or darker skin tones. Fluences cannot be compared across the different IPL systems; thus, it is

Name	Manufacturer	Optical spectrum (nm)	Available optical filters or handpieces	Spot sizes (mm²)
Lumenis One	Lumenis	515–1200	515, 560, 590, 615, 640, 695, 755	120, 525
StarLux 500 with LuxG handpiece	Palomar	500–670 & 870–1200	N/A	150
PhotoLight	Cynosure	400–1200	500, 560, 650	210, 460, 828
BBL	Sciton	420–1400	420, 515, 560, 590, 640, 695	225, 675

Table 11 Examples of commercially-available intense pulsed light systems used in the treatment of rosacea

recommended that they be set in accordance with manufacturer guidelines, frequently available in the form of presets or through on-screen menus.

Following a series of treatment, typically two to five sessions delivered every 4–6 weeks, an improvement of 20–83% in erythema of rosacea and 30–78% in telangiectasias may be achieved (Mark *et al.* 2003; Papageorgiou *et al.* 2008; Schroeter *et al.* 2005; Taub 2003) (**64, 65**). The incidence of flushing and inflammatory lesions has also been noted to decrease substantially (Taub 2003). Moreover, studies of cutaneous blood flow and objective color assessment have corroborated the associated clinical improvement in the symptoms and signs of rosacea (Kawana *et al.* 2007; Mark *et al.* 2003). The longevity of these effects has been evaluated in several studies and has been reported as 'at least 6 months' to over 3 years, depending on the study (Papageorgiou *et al.* 2008;

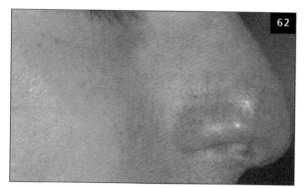
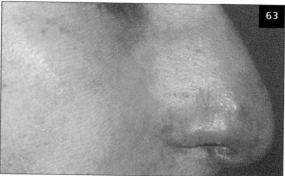

62, 63 Erythematotelangiectatic rosacea. 62 Before treatment. **63** Following five treatment sessions with an intense pulsed light source.

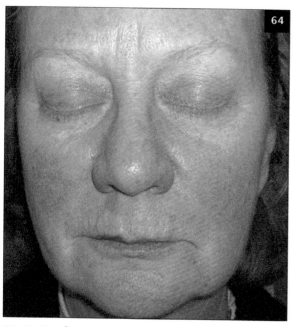
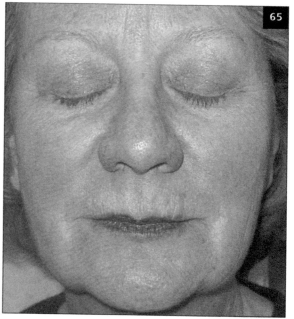

64, 65 Erythematotelangiectatic rosacea. 64 Before treatment. **65** Following five treatment sessions with an intense pulsed light source, showing very significant improvement in erythema.

Schroeter *et al*. 2005). As with the above discussion of PDL, we believe that the longevity of improvement depends, to a large extent, on the individual's continual exposure to rosacea triggers.

Adverse effects associated with the use of IPL systems in the treatment of rosacea are generally mild and short-lived. Mild-to-moderate erythema and edema are common and can last for 2–3 days. Purpura may occur, but is more common with lower-wavelength cut-off filters. Rectangular footprints corresponding to the IPL tip may become evident in individuals with sun tan, severely photodamaged skin, or those with darker skin tones. Caution must be exercised and higher-rated cut-off filters, multi-pulsed mode, and lower fluences are recommended in such patients. Blisters are uncommon and may at times be associated with a suboptimal choice of settings. These typically resolve without permanent sequelae and only rarely cause textural alterations (Schroeter *et al*. 2005; Sperber *et al*. 2005). Finally, since follicular melanin acts as a competing chromophore, treatment of skin covered with hair, such as the beard area in men, may result in temporary hair loss. This potentially-undesired effect is of special relevance during treatment with an IPL device, as most systems feature large spot sizes.

KTP AND Nd:YAG LASERS

While these lasers represent well-established therapeutic modalities for such vascular lesions as facial telangiectasias and leg veins, relatively little literature has been published on the use of these lasers specifically for rosacea.

At the core of both of these types of lasers is a Nd:YAG crystal that emits light with a wavelength of 1064 nm (*Table 12*). In a KTP laser, a potassium titanyl phosphate crystal is then used to double the frequency of light, thus halving its wavelength to 532 nm. The green light produced by the KTP laser is very near the oxyhemoglobin absorption peak of 542 nm and is, therefore, well absorbed by the target. In contrast, the infrared light emitted by the Nd:YAG laser falls within the broad yet relatively low oxyhemoglobin absorption band. This results in significantly lower absorption, requiring higher fluences to achieve substantial clinical effect. On the other hand, the longer wavelength is associated with much greater optical penetration depth into the dermis, allowing improved clearance of deeper vessels. Both systems are able to emit long pulses of laser

Name	Manufacturer	Wavelength (nm)	Cooling
DioLite^XP	Iridex	532	None
Aura-i	Iridex	532	None
Gemini	Iridex	532/1064	Contact
Cynergy	Cynosure	1064/595(PDL)	Air
Lyra-i	Iridex	1064	Contact
CoolGlide	Cutera	1064	Contact
Varia	CoolTouch	1064	Cryogen
GentleYAG	Candela	1064	Cryogen

Table 12 Examples of commercially-available Nd:YAG lasers, including KTP lasers

light, resulting in gradual heating of blood vessels without rupture of the vessel wall and subsequent purpura.

Very good or excellent improvement in facial telangiectasias following treatment with a KTP laser has been documented in several studies, with clearance rates as high as 94% reported after a single treatment (Cassuto *et al*. 2000; Clark *et al*. 2004). In our experience, however, several sessions (two to five) performed every 3–4 weeks are necessary for such impressive results (**66, 67**). In contrast, perialar telangiectasias are typically more resistant to treatment. Thus, after one KTP laser session, 53% of perialar telangiectasias showed good to excellent improvement (Goodman *et al*. 2002).

In a split-face comparison study, KTP laser was found to be more efficacious in eliminating telangiectasias and diffuse facial erythema compared to a 595 nm PDL used at subpurpuric doses. After three treatment sessions, clearance rates of 85% and 75% were achieved using the KTP laser and the PDL, respectively (Uebelhoer *et al*. 2007). Unfortunately, erythema and telangiectasias were not assessed separately in that study. On the other hand, a PDL may be somewhat more effective than a KTP laser in the improvement of facial telangiectasias when purpurogenic settings are employed (West & Alster 1998).

As mentioned above, light emitted by the 1064 nm Nd:YAG laser penetrates deeper into the dermis, thus reaching deeper vasculature. Moreover, since melanin absorption is low in the near-infrared portion of the

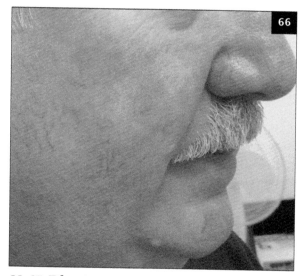
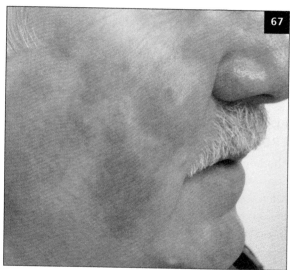

66, 67 Telangiectasia. 66 Before treatment. **67** Immediately after treatment with a KTP laser.

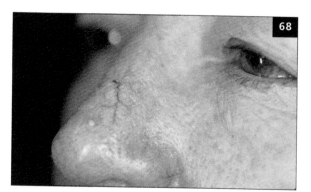
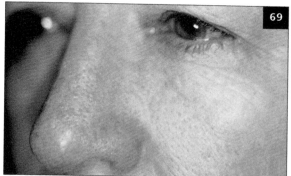

68, 69 Telangiectasia. 68 Before treatment. **69** After treatment with an Nd:YAG laser.

spectrum, this laser is also safer in darker-skinned individuals. On the other hand, because of higher absorption of light by water, treatments utilizing this wavelength are generally more painful compared to the PDL and the KTP laser. While the efficacy of Nd:YAG laser in the treatment of leg veins has been well documented, published reports on the use of this laser for facial telangiectasias have been very few. A study of facial telangiectasias and periorbital reticular veins treated with a 1064 nm Nd:YAG laser demonstrated greater than 75% improvement in nearly all patients after a single session (Eremia & Li 2002) (**68, 69**). Additional prospective studies are needed to

corroborate these findings, and to demonstrate the utility of these systems in the treatment of rosacea.

When telangiectatic blood vessels are treated with a KTP or an Nd:YAG laser, pulses are delivered without overlap with a clinical endpoint of immediate lightening or blanching of the target vessel. Pulse stacking should be avoided to prevent overheating and potential collateral damage, manifesting as white-gray discoloration of the overlying epidermis. In such cases, blistering and subsequent crusting are likely to occur, but generally resolve with local wound care in 5–7 days without long-term sequelae. Additional adverse effects are erythema and edema lasting 1–2 days, which may be more pronounced as compared to the PDL (Clark *et al.* 2004; Uebelhoer *et al.* 2007). On the other hand, atrophic scarring is relatively rare with these lasers; nonetheless, scarring is more frequent with the deep-penetrating light emitted by the 1064 nm Nd:YAG laser as compared to the other vascular-specific lasers.

FUTURE DIRECTIONS IN LIGHT-BASED TREATMENT OF ROSACEA

Photodynamic therapy (PDT) is a therapeutic modality approved in the US for the treatment of actinic keratoses, but also used off-label for various indications, including acne vulgaris and photorejuvenation. This procedure was extensively covered in Chapter 2 of this book. Recently, PDT utilizing either 5-aminolevulinic acid (ALA) or methyl aminolevulinate (MAL) has been employed for the treatment of recalcitrant cases of papulopustular rosacea. Long-term improvement has been anecdotally reported in several case reports and small studies following one to four sessions (Bryld & Jemec 2007; Katz & Patel 2006; Nybaek & Jemec 2005), although one additional small study failed to show significant improvement in rosacea (Togsverd-Bo *et al.* 2009). Thus, a potentially promising future therapeutic option, PDT use in the treatment of inflammatory rosacea needs to be evaluated in large prospective randomized studies.

8 LASERS AND SIMILAR DEVICES IN THE TREATMENT OF SEBACEOUS HYPERPLASIA

INTRODUCTION

AGING of the skin may be attributed to both intrinsic and extrinsic factors, with chronic exposure to ultraviolet (UV) radiation representing the greatest contributor to the latter group. As part of the pilosebaceous unit, sebaceous glands are cutaneous appendages that, likewise, undergo both intrinsic and extrinsic aging. Sebaceous hyperplasia is a benign glandular hyperproliferation that most often occurs on the face of middle-aged and elderly individuals. Although benign in its clinical behavior, sebaceous hyperplasia represents a significant cosmetic concern, especially when numerous. This chapter will present important clinical considerations, as well as the current data on the pathophysiology of sebaceous hyperplasia. It will then deal with laser- and light-based technologies and related procedures utilized in the treatment of these lesions.

AGING OF THE SEBACEOUS GLANDS AND THE PATHOPHYSIOLOGY OF SEBACEOUS HYPERPLASIA

Sebaceous glands form early in gestation as buds from the developing hair follicles (Holbrook *et al.* 1993). Although the number of these glands remains largely unchanged throughout life, their size changes based on the chronological age (Zouboulis & Boschnakow 2001). Well-developed in neonates, sebaceous glands then decrease in size and appear shrunken during infancy and childhood, only to enlarge, once again, during adrenarche and the subsequent puberty. Androgens appear to be the major determinant of both sebaceous gland development and sebum production; however, numerous other endocrine factors have been proposed to affect sebum production (Deplewski & Rosenfield 2000; Thody & Shuster 1989; Thiboutot *et al.* 2000; Zouboulis & Bohm 2004; Zouboulis *et al.* 2002). Sebum production remains largely unchanged until the eighth decade in men, while that in women starts to gradually decrease after menopause until a nadir in the seventh decade (Pochi *et al.* 1979).

Sebaceous glands secrete sebum in holocrine manner, with sebocyte disintegration and subsequent release of intracellular contents. As a result, glandular cells are completely renewed every month (Epstein & Epstein 1966). It has been suggested that cellular transition time–the time between germinative cell division and cellular disintegration–increases in the elderly, resulting in slower cellular turnover and eventual glandular hyperplasia (Plewig *et al.* 1971; Zouboulis & Boschnakow 2001). Cellular proliferation and mitotic activity within the sebaceous glands appear, once again, to be regulated (at least partially) by androgens, but not by estrogens (Ebling 1957, 1967; Sauter & Loud 1975). Such hyperproliferative effect may be dependent on gland localization, with facial sebocytes affected to a much greater extent as compared to nonfacial sites (Akamatsu *et al.* 1992). Additionally, insulin, thyroid-stimulating hormone, and hydrocortisone have also been found to up-regulate sebocyte proliferation (Zouboulis *et al.* 1998). Subsequent hyperplasia of undifferentiated sebaceous cells leads to the crowding and enlargement of glandular lobules, which, paradoxically, secrete very small amounts of sebum.

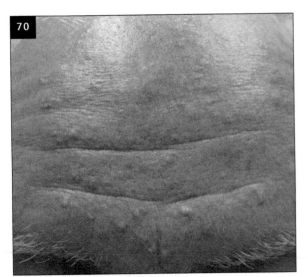

70 **Patient with numerous lesions of sebaceous hyperplasia** in association with extensive actinic damage.

Aside from these intrinsic factors, extrinsic factors, most notably UV radiation, have been shown to result in sebaceous gland hyperproliferation (**70**). Prolonged cumulative exposure to UV light causes sebaceous hyperplasia in hairless mice (Lesnik *et al.* 1992). Although UVB light was utilized in this study, the deeper-penetrating UVA rays may have a similar effect, but need to be further researched in the future (Zouboulis & Boschnakow 2001). In addition, long-term immunosuppression, especially with cyclosporine A and corticosteroids, following solid-organ transplants significantly increases the incidence of sebaceous gland hyperplasia (de Berker *et al.* 1996; Salim *et al.* 2006) (**71**). The exact mechanism of such an increase is unclear.

CLINICAL CONSIDERATIONS

The most common clinical presentation of sebaceous hyperplasia is that of a solitary or multiple yellowish papules, frequently with central umbilication around the follicular ostium and pearly appearance, thus most frequently resembling a basal cell carcinoma (**72**). Dermatoscopy is a useful tool in difficult cases, allowing for the differentiation between the yellow globules and peripheral wreath-like blood vessels of a sebaceous hyperplasia and the skin color and arborizing blood vessels of a basal cell carcinoma. A biopsy should be performed if clinical doubt persists.

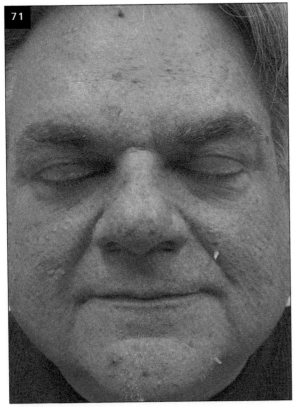

71 **Renal transplant recipient on life-long immunosuppression.** Notice the numerous lesions of sebaceous hyperplasia and incidental verrucae vulgares.

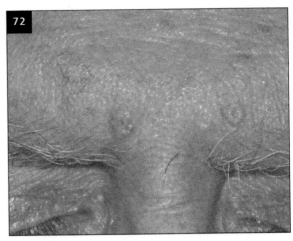

72 **Sebaceous hyperplasia** clinically resembling a basal cell carcinoma.

While most lesions occur in middle-aged individuals, premature appearance has been documented in patients as early as 12 years of age (De Villez & Roberts 1982; Grimalt et al. 1997). Additionally, familial involvement with autosomal dominant inheritance has also been documented (Boonchai & Leenutaphong 1997; Dupre et al. 1983). In such cases, a diagnosis of Muir–Torre syndrome, characterized by multiple benign and malignant sebaceous neoplasms, keratoacanthoma-like lesions, and internal malignancies, must be considered (Schwartz & Torre 1995).

With a recent finding of a significantly increased incidence of nonmelanoma skin cancer in renal transplant patients with lesions of sebaceous hyperplasia as compared to those without sebaceous hyperplasia, these benign glandular hyperproliferations may actually become an important prognostic marker in this population (Salim et al. 2006). However, this finding needs to be confirmed in additional prospective studies.

LASERS AND SIMILAR TECHNOLOGIES IN THE TREATMENT OF SEBACEOUS HYPERPLASIA

Traditional destructive modalities used in the treatment of sebaceous hyperplasia include cryosurgery, electrodessication, curettage, and topical bi- and trichloracetic acid (Bader & Scarborough 2000; Rosian et al. 1991; Wheeland & Wiley 1987). These therapies may at times, however, be associated with prolonged dyschromia and scarring. Additionally, oral isotretinoin has been shown to be very effective in the treatment of these lesions, but is associated with multiple adverse effects, as well as rapid recurrence following the discontinuation of therapy (Burton & Sawchuk 1985; Grekin & Ellis 1984; Grimalt et al. 1997). On the other hand, several lasers and light-based procedures have been used with success to deliver target-specific treatment with long-term improvement and few or no long-term adverse effects (Table 13).

Although effective in a pilot study, the argon laser delivers nonspecific coagulation and, therefore, a higher risk of complications (Landthaler et al. 1984). More recently, a pulsed-dye laser (PDL) has been used in the treatment of these lesions. The tissue target for this laser appears to be the blood vessels that surround the

Oral isotretinoin
Cryosurgery
Electrodessication
Curettage
Bi- and trichloracetic acid
Lasers
Pulsed-dye laser
Mid-infrared lasers
Photodynamic therapy

Table 13 Therapeutic modalities commonly used in the treatment of sebaceous hyperplasia

sebaceous duct ostium (Aghassi et al. 2000). In the studies, a 585-nm laser was used with traditional, purpurogenic settings as described in Chapter 7 of this book. One to three sessions were required to clear the majority of lesions, although the risk of partial or complete recurrence following a single session was 35% in one of the studies (Aghassi et al. 2000; Schonermark et al. 1997).

As mentioned in Chapters 3 and 4, mid-infrared lasers emit light, whose wavelength penetrates deep into the dermis and is preferentially absorbed by water. Bulk heating of the dermal water content appears to alter sebaceous gland function and, possibly, structure. In one study, thermal coagulation of the sebaceous lobule was demonstrated in rabbit and human skin immediately following laser irradiation (Paithankar et al. 2002). By extension, a 1,450-nm diode laser has been used successfully in the treatment of sebaceous hyperplasia. In a small study of 10 patients, high fluences of up to 17 J/cm² were used in combination with prolonged cooling time to achieve excellent improvement in 70% of patients after one to five treatment sessions (No et al. 2004). Following treatment, the individual lesions may form crusts and demonstrate oily discharge for up to 3 days, with complete healing typically achieved by 1 week. Although adverse effects were rare, transient dyschromia and atrophic scarring were noted in one patient each. In our practice, we tend to utilize lower fluences in combination with stacked pulses and multiple treatment sessions. Larger studies are needed to evaluate for the optimal treatment parameters, the success rate, and the persistence of improvement.

The most extensively studied light-based treatment modality for the treatment of sebaceous hyperplasia is photodynamic therapy (PDT). Target specificity is achieved by the preferential uptake of the photosensitizing compounds by the sebaceous glands (Divaris *et al.* 1990; Hongcharu *et al.* 2000). The complete mechanism of action of PDT is described at length in Chapter 3.

Both 5-aminolevulinic acid (ALA) and methyl aminolevulinate (MAL) have been used for this indication (Horio *et al.* 2003; Perrett *et al.* 2006). Although the first report utilized an ALA incubation time of 4 hours, subsequent studies shortened the incubation period to 1 hour or less without a perceptible decrease in efficacy (Alster & Tanzi 2003; Goldman 2003; Horio *et al.* 2003). Likewise, various lasers and light sources have been used to activate the topical photosensitizers, including PDL, blue and red noncohesive lights, intense pulsed light (IPL) sources, and even a halogen bulb of a simple slide projector (Alster & Tanzi 2003; Gold *et al.* 2004; Goldman 2003; Horio *et al.* 2003; Richey & Hopson 2004). Although not definitively proven, ALA activation using a PDL with stacked pulses may result in faster clearance, necessitating one to two sessions, as compared to the other sources of light, which typically require two to six treatment sessions administered monthly (Alster & Tanzi 2003; Horio *et al.* 2003; Richey & Hopson 2004).

Although the initial clearance rates are high, variably reported at 53–100% following multiple sessions, up to 20% of lesions recurred in one study within 3–4 months (Richey & Hopson 2004). Other studies documented a persistence of clearance throughout the follow-up period of up to 12 months (Horio *et al.* 2003). Thus, the need for maintenance therapy has not yet been firmly established. Adverse effects are similar to those encountered in the treatment of acne using PDT and typically include transient erythema and edema, focal crusting, and, less commonly, blistering and postinflammatory hyperpigmentation, especially in individuals with darker skin tones.

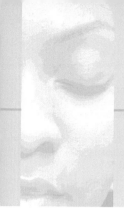

REFERENCES

Chapter 1

Adebamowo CA, Spiegelman D, Danby FW, Frazier AL, Willett WC, Holmes MD (2005). High school dietary dairy intake and teenage acne. *Journal of the American Academy of Dermatology* **52**(2):207–214.

Aizawa H, Nakada Y, Niimura M (1995). Androgen status in adolescent women with acne vulgaris. *Journal of Dermatology* **22**(7):530–532.

Aizawa H, Niimura M (1995). Elevated serum insulin-like growth factor-1 (IGF-1) levels in women with postadolescent acne. *Journal of Dermatology* **22**(4):249–252.

Anderson PC (1971). Foods as the cause of acne. *American Family Physician* **3**(3):102–103.

Baker BS, Ovigne JM, Powles AV, Corcoran S, Fry L (2003). Normal keratinocytes express Toll-like receptors (TLRs) 1, 2 and 5: modulation of TLR expression in chronic plaque psoriasis. *British Journal of Dermatology* **148**(4):670–679.

Bataille V, Snieder H, MacGregor AJ, Sasieni P, Spector TD (2002). The influence of genetics and environmental factors in the pathogenesis of acne: a twin study of acne in women. *Journal of Investigative Dermatology* **119**(6):1317–1322.

Bershad S (2003). The unwelcome return of the acne diet. *Archives of Dermatology* **139**:940–941.

Bershad SV (2005). Diet and acne–slim evidence, again. *Journal of the American Academy of Dermatology* **52**:1102.

Berson DS, Chalker DK, Harper JC, Leyden JJ, Shalita AR, Webster GF (2003). Current concepts in the treatment of acne: report from a clinical roundtable. *Cutis* **72**(1 Suppl):5–13.

Burke BM, Cunliffe WJ (1984). The assessment of acne vulgaris–the Leeds technique. *British Journal of Dermatology* **111**(1):83–92.

Burkhart CG, Burkhart CN (2006). Genome sequence of *Propionibacterium acnes* reveals immunogenic and surface-associated genes confirming existence of the acne biofilm. *International Journal of Dermatology* **45**(7):872.

Burkhart CG, Burkhart CN (2007). Expanding the microcomedone theory and acne therapeutics: *Propionibacterium acnes* biofilm produces biological glue that holds corneocytes together to form plug. *Journal of the American Academy of Dermatology* **57**(4):722–724.

Cappel M, Mauger D, Thiboutot D (2005). Correlation between serum levels of insulin-like growth factor 1, dehydroepiandrosterone sulfate, and dihydrotestosterone and acne lesion counts in adult women. *Archives of Dermatology* **141**(3):333–338.

Chen W, Thiboutot D, Zouboulis CC (2002). Cutaneous androgen metabolism: basic research and clinical perspectives. *Journal of Investigative Dermatology* **119**(5):992–1007.

Child FJ, Fuller LC, Higgins EM, Du Vivier AW (1999). A study of the spectrum of skin disease occurring in a black population in south-east London. *British Journal of Dermatology* **141**(3):512–517.

Christiansen J, Holm P, Reymann F (1976). Treatment of acne vulgaris with the retinoic acid derivative Ro 11-1430. A controlled clinical trial against retinoic acid. *Dermatologica* **153**(3):172–176.

Chuh AA, Zawar V, Wong WC, Lee A (2004). The association of smoking and acne in men in Hong Kong and in India: a retrospective case–control study in primary care settings. *Clinical and Experimental Dermatology* **29**(6):597–599.

Collier CN, Harper JC, Cantrell WC, Wang W, Foster KW, Elewski BE (2008). The prevalence of acne in adults 20 years and older. *Journal of the American Academy of Dermatology* **58**(1):56–59.

Cook CH, Centner RL, Michaels SE (1979). An acne grading method using photographic standards. *Archives of Dermatology* **115**(5):571–575.

Cordain L (2005). Implications for the role of diet in acne. *Seminars in Cutaneous Medicine and Surgery* **24**:84–91.

Cordain L, Lindeberg S, Hurtado M, Hill K, Eaton SB, Brand-Miller J (2002). Acne vulgaris: a disease of Western civilization. *Archives of Dermatology* **138**(12):1584–1590.

Cunliffe WJ, Gould DJ (1979). Prevalence of facial acne vulgaris in late adolescence and in adults. *British Medical Journal* **1**(6171):1109–1110.

Cunliffe WJ, Baron SE, Coulson IH (2001). A clinical and therapeutic study of 29 patients with infantile acne. *British Journal of Dermatology* **145**(3):463–466.

Danby FW (2005). Acne and milk, the diet myth, and beyond. *Journal of the American Academy of Dermatology* **52**(2):360–362.

Doshi A, Zaheer A, Stiller MJ (1997). A comparison of current acne grading systems and proposal of a novel system. *International Journal of Dermatology* **36**(6):416–418.

Downing DT, Stewart ME, Wertz PW, Strauss JS (1986). Essential fatty acids and acne. *Journal of the American Academy of Dermatology* **14**(2 Pt 1):221–225.

Evans DM, Kirk KM, Nyholt DR, Novac C, Martin NG (2005). Teenage acne is influenced by genetic factors. *British Journal of Dermatology* **152**(3):579–581.

Firooz A, Sarhangnejad R, Davoudi SM, Nassiri-Kashani M (2005). Acne and smoking: is there a relationship? *BMC Dermatology* **5**:2.

Friedman GD (1984). Twin studies of disease heritability based on medical records: application to acne vulgaris. *Acta Geneticae Medicae Gemellologiae* **33**(3):487–495.

Fritsch M, Orfanos CE, Zouboulis CC (2001). Sebocytes are the key regulators of androgen homeostasis in human skin. *Journal of Investigative Dermatology* **116**(5):793–800.

Fulton JE Jr, Plewig G, Kligman AM (1969). Effect of chocolate on acne vulgaris. *Journal of the American Medical Association* **210**(11):2071–2074.

Goh CL, Akarapanth R (1994). Epidemiology of skin disease among children in a referral skin clinic in Singapore. *Pediatric Dermatology* **11**(2):125–128.

Goulden V, Clark SM, Cunliffe WJ (1997). Post-adolescent acne: a review of clinical features. *British Journal of Dermatology* **136**(1):66–70.

Goulden V, McGeown CH, Cunliffe WJ (1999). The familial risk of adult acne: a comparison between first-degree relatives of affected and unaffected individuals. *British Journal of Dermatology* **141**(2):297–300.

Guy R, Green MR, Kealey T (1996). Modeling acne *in vitro*. *Journal of Investigative Dermatology* **106**(1):176–182.

Halder RM, Grimes PE, McLaurin CI, Kress MA, Kenney JA Jr (1983). Incidence of common dermatoses in a predominantly black dermatologic practice. *Cutis* **32**(4):388–390.

Halder RM, Holmes YC, Bridgeman-Shah S, Kligman AM (1996). A clinicopathological study of acne vulgaris in black females. *Journal of Investigative Dermatology* **106**:888.

Hoeffler U (1977). Enzymatic and hemolytic properties of *Propionibacterium acnes* and related bacteria. *Journal of Clinical Microbiology* **6**(6):555–558.

Imperato-McGinley J, Gautier T, Cai L Q, Yee B, Epstein J, Pochi P (1993). The androgen control of sebum production. Studies of subjects with dihydrotestosterone deficiency and complete androgen insensitivity. *Journal of Clinical Endocrinology and Metabolism* 76(2):524–528.

Ingham E, Holland KT, Gowland G, Cunliffe WJ (1980). Purification and partial characterization of an acid phosphatase (EC 3.1.3.2) produced by *Propionibacterium acnes. Journal of General Microbiology* 118(1):59–65.

Ingham E, Holland KT, Gowland G, Cunliffe WJ (1981). Partial purification and characterization of lipase (EC 3.1.1.3) from *Propionibacterium acnes. Journal of General Microbiology* 124(2):393–401.

James KW, Tisserand JB Jr (1958). Treatment of acne vulgaris. *GP* 18(3):130–139.

Jansen T, Plewig G (1998). Acne fulminans. *International Journal of Dermatology* 37(4):254–257.

Jansen T, Burgdorf WH, Plewig G (1997). Pathogenesis and treatment of acne in childhood. *Pediatric Dermatology* 14(1):17–21.

Jemec GB, Linneberg A, Nielsen NH, Frolund L, Madsen F, Jorgensen T (2002). Have oral contraceptives reduced the prevalence of acne? A population-based study of acne vulgaris, tobacco smoking and oral contraceptives. *Dermatology* 204(3):179–184.

Kamisango K, Saiki I, Tanio Y, *et al.* (1982). Structures and biological activities of peptidoglycans of *Listeria monocytogenes* and *Propionibacterium acnes. Journal of Biochemistry* 92(1):23–33.

Kang S, Cho S, Chung JH, Hammerberg C, Fisher GJ, Voorhees JJ (2005). Inflammation and extracellular matrix degradation mediated by activated transcription factors nuclear factor-kappaB and activator protein-1 in inflammatory acne lesions *in vivo. American Journal of Pathology* 166(6):1691–1699.

Kaymak Y, Adisen E, Ilter N, Bideci A, Gurler D, Celik B (2007). Dietary glycemic index and glucose, insulin, insulin-like growth factor-1, insulin-like growth factor binding protein 3, and leptin levels in patients with acne. *Journal of the American Academy of Dermatology* 57(5):819–823.

Kim J, Ochoa MT, Krutzik SR, *et al.* (2002). Activation of toll-like receptor 2 in acne triggers inflammatory cytokine responses. *Journal of Immunology* 169(3):1535–1541.

Klaz I, Kochba I, Shohat T, Zarka S, Brenner S (2006). Severe acne vulgaris and tobacco smoking in young men. *Journal of Investigative Dermatology* 126(8):1749–1752.

Knaggs HE, Holland DB, Morris C, Wood EJ, Cunliffe WJ (1994a). Quantification of cellular proliferation in acne using the monoclonal antibody Ki-67. *Journal of Investigative Dermatology* 102(1):89–92.

Knaggs HE, Hughes BR, Morris C, Wood EJ, Holland DB, Cunliffe WJ (1994b). Immunohistochemical study of desmosomes in acne vulgaris. *British Journal of Dermatology* 130(6):731–737.

Kraning KK, Odland GF (1979). Prevalence, morbidity and cost of dermatologic diseases. *Journal of Investigative Dermatology* 73:395–513.

Lee MR, Cooper A (2006). Acne vulgaris in monozygotic twins. *Australasian Journal of Dermatology* 47(2):145.

Leyden JJ, McGinley KJ, Mills OH, Kligman AM (1975). *Propionibacterium* levels in patients with and without acne vulgaris. *Journal of Investigative Dermatology* 65(4):382–384.

Leyden JJ, McGinley KJ, Vowels B (1998). *Propionibacterium acnes* colonization in acne and nonacne. *Dermatology* 196(1):55–58.

Logan AC (2003). Omega-3 fatty acids and acne. *Archives of Dermatology* 139:941–942.

Lowenstein EJ (2006). Diagnosis and management of the dermatologic manifestations of the polycystic ovary syndrome. *Dermatologic Therapy* 19(4):210–223.

Lucky AW, McGuire J, Rosenfield RL, Lucky PA, Rich BH (1983). Plasma androgens in women with acne vulgaris. *Journal of Investigative Dermatology* 81(1):70–74.

Lucky AW, Biro FM, Huster GA, Leach AD, Morrison JA, Ratterman J (1994). Acne vulgaris in premenarchal girls. An early sign of puberty associated with rising levels of dehydroepiandrosterone. *Archives of Dermatology* 130(3):308–314.

Lucky AW, Barber BL, Girman CJ, *et al.* (1996). A multirater validation study to assess the reliability of acne lesion counting. *Journal of the American Academy of Dermatology* 35(4):559–565.

Lucky AW (1998). A review of infantile and pediatric acne. *Dermatology* 196(1):95–97.

Mann MW, Ellis SS, Mallory SB (2007). Infantile acne as the initial sign of an adrenocortical tumor. *Journal of the American Academy of Dermatology* 56(2 Suppl):S15–S18.

Marynick SP, Chakmakjian ZH, McCaffree DL, Herndon JH Jr (1983). Androgen excess in cystic acne. *New England Journal of Medicine* 308(17):981–986.

Menon GK, Feingold KR, Moser AH, Brown BE, Elias PM (1985). *De novo* sterologenesis in the skin. II. Regulation by cutaneous barrier requirements. *Journal of Lipid Research* 26(4):418–427.

Michaelson G, Juhlin L, Vahlquist A (1977). Oral zinc sulphate therapy for acne vulgaris. *Acta Dermato-Venereologica* 57(4):372.

Mills CM, Peters TJ, Finlay AY (1993). Does smoking influence acne? *Clinical and Experimental Dermatology* 18(2):100–101.

Mourelatos K, Eady EA, Cunliffe WJ, Clark SM, Cove JH (2007). Temporal changes in sebum excretion and propionibacterial colonization in preadolescent children with and without acne. *British Journal of Dermatology* 156(1):22–31.

Nagy I, Pivarcsi A, Koreck A, Szell M, Urban E, Kemeny L (2005). Distinct strains of *Propionibacterium acnes* induce selective human beta-defensin-2 and interleukin-8 expression in human keratinocytes through toll-like receptors. *Journal of Investigative Dermatology* 124(5):931–938.

New MI, Wilson RC (1999). Steroid disorders in children: congenital adrenal hyperplasia and apparent mineralocorticoid excess. *Proceedings of the National Academy of Sciences of the United States of America* 96(22):12790–12797.

Phillips SB, Kollias N, Gillies R, *et al.* (1997). Polarized light photography enhances visualization of inflammatory lesions of acne vulgaris. *Journal of the American Academy of Dermatology* 37(6):948–952.

Pillsbury DM, Shelley WB, Kligman AM (1956). *Dermatology.* Saunders, Philadelphia.

Pivarcsi A, Bodai L, Rethi B, *et al.* (2003). Expression and function of Toll-like receptors 2 and 4 in human keratinocytes. *International Immunology* 15(6):721–730.

Plewig G, Kligman AM (1975). Classification of acne vulgaris. In: *Acne: Morphogenesis and Treatment*. Springer-Verlag, New York, pp. 162–163.

Poli F, Dreno B, Verschoore M (2001). An epidemiological study of acne in female adults: results of a survey conducted in France. *Journal of the European Academy of Dermatology and Venereology* 15(6):541–545.

Puhvel SM, Reisner RM (1972). The production of hyaluronidase (hyaluronate lyase) by *Corynebacterium acnes. Journal of Investigative Dermatology* 58(2):66–70.

Rombouts S, Nijsten T, Lambert J (2007). Cigarette smoking and acne in adolescents: results from a cross-sectional study. *Journal of the European Academy of Dermatology and Venereology* 21(3):326–333.

Sawaya ME, Price VH (1997). Different levels of 5alpha-reductase type I and II, aromatase, and androgen receptor in hair follicles of women and men with androgenetic alopecia. *Journal of Investigative Dermatology* 109(3):296–300.

Schaefer O (1971). When the Eskimo comes to town. *Nutrition Today* 6:8–16.

Schafer T, Nienhaus A, Vieluf D, Berger J, Ring J (2001). Epidemiology of acne in the general population: the risk of smoking. *British Journal of Dermatology* 145(1):100–104.

Schaller M, Loewenstein M, Borelli C, *et al.* (2005). Induction of a chemoattractive proinflammatory cytokine response after stimulation of keratinocytes with *Propionibacterium acnes* and coproporphyrin III. *British Journal of Dermatology* **153**(1):66–71.

Seukeran DC, Cunliffe WJ (1999). The treatment of acne fulminans: a review of 25 cases. *British Journal of Dermatology* **141**(2):307–309.

Shalita AR, Leyden JJ Jr, Kligman AM (1997). Reliability of acne lesion counting. *Journal of the American Academy of Dermatology* **37**(4):672.

Smith RN, Mann NJ, Braue A, Makelainen H, Varigos GA (2007). The effect of a high-protein, low glycemic-load diet versus a conventional, high glycemic-load diet on biochemical parameters associated with acne vulgaris: a randomized, investigator-masked, controlled trial. *Journal of the American Academy of Dermatology* **57**(2):247–256.

Smythe CD, Greenall M, Kealey T (1998). The activity of HMG-CoA reductase and acetyl-CoA carboxylase in human apocrine sweat glands, sebaceous glands, and hair follicles is regulated by phosphorylation and by exogenous cholesterol. *Journal of Investigative Dermatology* **111**(1):139–48.

Steiner PE (1946). Necropsies on Okinawans: anatomic and pathologic observations. *Archives of Pathology* **42**:359–380.

Stern RS (1992). The prevalence of acne on the basis of physical examination. *Journal of the American Academy of Dermatology* **26**(6):931–935.

Stewart ME, Downing DT, Cook JS, Hansen JR, Strauss JS (1992). Sebaceous gland activity and serum dehydroepiandrosterone sulfate levels in boys and girls. *Archives of Dermatology* **128**(10):1345–1348.

Stratakis CA, Mastorakos G, Mitsiades NS, Mitsiades CS, Chrousos GP (1998). Skin manifestations of Cushing disease in children and adolescents before and after the resolution of hypercortisolemia. *Pediatric Dermatology* **15**(4):253–258.

Strauss JS, Pochi PE (1964). Effect of cyclic progestin-estrogen therapy on sebum and acne in women. *Journal of the American Medical Association* **190**(9):815–819.

Strauss JS, Krowchuk DP, Leyden JJ, *et al.* (2007). Guidelines of care for acne vulgaris management. *Journal of the American Academy of Dermatology* **56**(4):651–663.

Takeda K, Akira S (2004). Microbial recognition by Toll-like receptors. *Journal of Dermatological Science* **34**(2):73–82.

The Rotterdam ESHRE/ASRM-Sponsored PCOS consensus workshop group 2004. Revised 2003 consensus on diagnostic criteria and long-term health risks related to polycystic ovary syndrome (PCOS). *Human Reproduction* **19**(1):41–47.

Thiboutot D, Harris G, Iles V, Cimis G, Gilliland K, Hagari S (1995). Activity of the type 1 5 alpha-reductase exhibits regional differences in isolated sebaceous glands and whole skin. *Journal of Investigative Dermatology* **105**(2):209–214.

Thiboutot D, Sivarajah A, Gilliland K, Cong Z, Clawson G (2000). The melanocortin 5 receptor is expressed in human sebaceous glands and rat preputial cells. *Journal of Investigative Dermatology* **115**(4):614–619.

Treloar V (2003). Diet and acne redux. *Archives of Dermatology* **139**:941.

Treloar V, Logan AC, Danby FW, Cordain L, Mann NJ (2008). Comment on acne and glycemic index. *Journal of the American Academy of Dermatology* **58**(1):175–177.

Trivedi NR, Gilliland KL, Zhao W, Liu W, Thiboutot DM (2006). Gene array expression profiling in acne lesions reveals marked upregulation of genes involved in inflammation and matrix remodeling. *Journal of Investigative Dermatology* **126**(5):1071–1079.

Voorhees JJ, Wilkins JW Jr, Hayes E, Harrell ER (1972). Nodulocystic acne as a phenotypic feature of the XYY genotype. *Archives of Dermatology* **105**(6):913–919.

Vowels BR, Yang S, Leyden JJ (1995). Induction of proinflammatory cytokines by a soluble factor of *Propionibacterium acnes*: implications for chronic inflammatory acne. *Infection and Immunity* **63**(8):3158–3165.

White GM (1998). Recent findings in the epidemiologic evidence, classification, and subtypes of acne vulgaris. *Journal of the American Academy of Dermatology* **39**(2 Pt 3):S34–37.

Whitmarsh AJ, Davis RJ (1996). Transcription factor AP-1 regulation by mitogen-activated protein kinase signal transduction pathways. *Journal of Molecular Medicine* **74**(10):589–607.

Wilkins JW Jr, Voorhees JJ (1970). Prevalence of nodulocystic acne in white and Negro males. *Archives of Dermatology* **102**(6):631–634.

Witkowski JA, Simons HM (1966). Objective evaluation of demethylchlortetracycline hydrochloride in the treatment of acne. *Journal of the American Medical Association* **196**(5):397–400.

Witkowski JA, Parish LC (1999). From other ghosts of the past: acne lesion counting. *Journal of the American Academy of Dermatology* **40**(1):131.

Zouboulis CC, Bohm M (2004). Neuroendocrine regulation of sebocytes–a pathogenetic link between stress and acne. *Experimental Dermatology* **13**(4 Suppl):31–35.

Zouboulis CC, Seltmann H, Hiroi N, *et al.* (2002). Corticotropin-releasing hormone: an autocrine hormone that promotes lipogenesis in human sebocytes. *Proceedings of the National Academy of Sciences of the United States of America* **99**(10):7148–7153.

Chapter 2

Abergel RP, Meeker CA, Oikarinen H, Oikarinen AI, Uitto J (1985). Retinoid modulation of connective tissue metabolism in keloid fibroblast cultures. *Archives of Dermatology* **121**(5):632–635.

Agwuh KN, MacGowan A (2006). Pharmacokinetics and pharmacodynamics of the tetracyclines including glycylcyclines. *Journal of Antimicrobial Chemotherapy* **58**(2):256–265.

Akman A, Durusoy C, Senturk M, Koc CK, Soyturk D, Alpsoy E (2007). Treatment of acne with intermittent and conventional isotretinoin: a randomized, controlled multicenter study. *Archives of Dermatological Research* **299**(10):467–473.

Alcalay J, Landau M, Zucker A (2001). Analysis of laboratory data in acne patients treated with isotretinoin: is there really a need to perform routine laboratory tests? *Journal of Dermatological Treatment* **12**(1):9–12.

Allec J, Chatelus A, Wagner N (1997). Skin distribution and pharmaceutical aspects of adapalene gel. *Journal of the American Academy of Dermatology* **36**(6 Pt 2):S119–S125.

Allen JG, Bloxham DP (1989). The pharmacology and pharmacokinetics of the retinoids. *Pharmacology and Therapeutics* **40**(1):1–27.

Amichai B, Shemer A, Grunwald MH (2006). Low-dose isotretinoin in the treatment of acne vulgaris. *Journal of the American Academy of Dermatology* **54**(4):644–646.

Amin AR, Attur MG, Thakker GD, *et al.* (1996). A novel mechanism of action of tetracyclines: effects on nitric oxide synthases. *Proceedings of the National Academy of Sciences of the United States of America* **93**(24):14014–14019.

Angeloni VL, Salasche SJ, Ortiz R (1987). Nail, skin, and scleral pigmentation induced by minocycline. *Cutis* **40**(3):229–233.

Aragona P, Cannavo SP, Borgia F, Guarneri F (2005). Utility of studying the ocular surface in patients with acne vulgaris treated with oral isotretinoin: a randomized controlled trial. *British Journal of Dermatology* **152**(3):576–578.

Aygun C, Kocaman O, Gurbuz Y, Senturk O, Hulagu S (2007). Clindamycin-induced acute cholestatic hepatitis. *World Journal of Gastroenterology* **13**(40):5408–5410.

Azurdia RM, Sharpe GR (1999). Isotretinoin treatment for acne vulgaris and its cutaneous and ocular side-effects. *British Journal of Dermatology* **141**(5):947.

Barth JH, Macdonald-Hull SP, Mark J, Jones RG, Cunliffe WJ (1993). Isotretinoin therapy for acne vulgaris: a re-evaluation of the need for measurements of plasma lipids and liver function tests. *British Journal of Dermatology* **129**(6):704–707.

Barza M, Goldstein JA, Kane A, Feingold DS, Pochi PE (1982). Systemic absorption of clindamycin hydrochloride after topical application. *Journal of the American Academy of Dermatology* 7(2):208–214.

Becker LE, Bergstresser PR, Whiting DA, *et al*. (1981). Topical clindamycin therapy for acne vulgaris. A cooperative clinical study. *Archives of Dermatology* 117(8):482–485.

Berger R, Barba A, Fleischer A, *et al*. (2007). A double-blinded, randomized, vehicle-controlled, multicenter, parallel-group study to assess the safety and efficacy of tretinoin gel microsphere 0.04% in the treatment of acne vulgaris in adults. *Cutis* 80(2):152–157.

Bernstein LJ, Geronemus RG (1997). Keloid formation with the 585-nm pulsed dye laser during isotretinoin treatment. *Archives of Dermatology* 133(1):111–112.

Beylot C, Doutre MS, Beylot-Barry M (1998). Oral contraceptives and cyproterone acetate in female acne treatment. *Dermatology* 196(1):148–152.

Bihorac A, Ozener C, Akoglu E, Kullu S (1999). Tetracycline-induced acute interstitial nephritis as a cause of acute renal failure. *Nephron* 81(1):72–75.

Bladon PT, Burke BM, Cunliffe WJ, Forster RA, Holland KT, King K (1986). Topical azelaic acid and the treatment of acne: a clinical and laboratory comparison with oral tetracycline. *British Journal of Dermatology* 114(4):493–499.

Bojar RA, Holland KT, Cunliffe WJ (1991). The *in-vitro* antimicrobial effects of azelaic acid upon *Propionibacterium acnes* strain P37. *Journal of Antimicrobial Chemotherapy* 28(6):843–853.

Bojar RA, Cunliffe WJ, Holland KT (1994). Disruption of the transmembrane pH gradient–a possible mechanism for the antibacterial action of azelaic acid in *Propionibacterium acnes* and *Staphylococcus* epidermidis. *Journal of Antimicrobial Chemotherapy* 34(3):321–330.

Boudou P, Chivot M, Vexiau P, *et al*. (1994). Evidence for decreased androgen 5 alpha-reduction in skin and liver of men with severe acne after 13-cis-retinoic acid treatment. *Journal of Clinical Endocrinology and Metabolism* 78(5):1064–1069.

Boudou P, Soliman H, Chivot M, *et al*. (1995). Effect of oral isotretinoin treatment on skin androgen receptor levels in male acneic patients. *Journal of Clinical Endocrinology and Metabolism* 80(4):1158–1161.

Bozkurt B, Irkec MT, Atakan N, Orhan M, Geyik PO (2002). Lacrimal function and ocular complications in patients treated with systemic isotretinoin. *European Journal of Ophthalmology* 12(3):173–176.

Bubalo JS, Blasdel CS, Bearden DT (2003). Neutropenia after single-dose clindamycin for dental prophylaxis. *Pharmacotherapy* 23(1):101–103.

Burke B, Eady EA, Cunliffe WJ (1983). Benzoyl peroxide versus topical erythromycin in the treatment of acne vulgaris. *British Journal of Dermatology* 108(2):199–204.

Burke BM, Cunliffe WJ (1985). Oral spironolactone therapy for female patients with acne, hirsutism or androgenic alopecia. *British Journal of Dermatology* 112(1):124–125.

Campbell JE, Carter WH (2005). Comments on the important drug interaction of warfarin and sulfamethoxazole. *Archives of Internal Medicine* 165(21):2540.

Carr BR, Ory H (1997). Estrogen and progestin components of oral contraceptives: relationship to vascular disease. *Contraception* 55(5):267–272.

Chan TY (1997). Co-trimoxazole-induced severe haemolysis: the experience of a large general hospital in Hong Kong. *Pharmacoepidemiology and Drug Safety* 6(2):89–92.

Chandraratna RA (1996). Tazarotene–first of a new generation of receptor-selective retinoids. *British Journal of Dermatology* 135(49 Suppl):18–25.

Chia CY, Lane W, Chibnall J, Allen A, Siegfried E (2005). Isotretinoin therapy and mood changes in adolescents with moderate to severe acne: a cohort study. *Archives of Dermatology* 141(5):557–560.

Chivot M (2001) Acne flare-up and deterioration with oral isotretinoin. *Annals of Dermatology and Venereology* 128(3 Pt 1):224–228.

Coenen CM, Thomas CM, Borm GF, Hollanders JM, Rolland R (1996). Changes in androgens during treatment with four low-dose contraceptives. *Contraception* 53(3):171–176.

Cogliano V, Grosse Y, Baan R, *et al*. (2005). Carcinogenicity of combined oestrogen-progestagen contraceptives and menopausal treatment. *Lancet Oncology* 6(8):552–553.

Crokaert F, Hubloux A, Cauchie P (1998). A Phase I determination of azithromycin in plasma during a 6-week period in normal volunteers after a standard dose of 500 mg once daily for 3 days. *Clinical Drug Investigation* 16(2):161–166.

Cunliffe WJ, Stainton C, Forster RA (1983). Topical benzoyl peroxide increases the sebum excretion rate in patients with acne. *British Journal of Dermatology* 109(5):577–579.

Cunliffe WJ, Poncet M, Loesche C, Verschoore M (1998). A comparison of the efficacy and tolerability of adapalene 0.1% gel versus tretinoin 0.025% gel in patients with acne vulgaris: a meta-analysis of five randomized trials. *British Journal of Dermatology* 139(52 Suppl):48–56.

Cunliffe WJ, Aldana OL, Goulden V (1999). Oral trimethoprim: a relatively safe and successful third-line treatment for acne vulgaris. *British Journal of Dermatology* 141(4):757–758.

D'Addario SF, Bryan ME, Stringer WA, Johnson SM (2003). Minocycline-induced immune thrombocytopenia presenting as Schamberg's disease. *Journal of Drugs in Dermatology* 2(3):320–323.

Danielson DA, Jick H, Hunter JR, Stergachis A, Madsen S (1982). Nonestrogenic drugs and breast cancer. *American Journal of Epidemiology* 116(2):329–332.

Darwiche N, Bazzi H, El-Touni L, *et al*. (2005). Regulation of ultraviolet B radiation-mediated activation of AP1 signaling by retinoids in primary keratinocytes. *Radiation Research* 163(3):296–306.

Del Rosso J (2008). Emerging topical antimicrobial options for mild-to-moderate acne: a review of the clinical evidence. *Journal of Drugs in Dermatology* 7(2Suppl):S2–S7.

Dickinson BD, Altman RD, Nielsen NH, Sterling ML (2001). Drug interactions between oral contraceptives and antibiotics. *Obstetrics and Gynecology* 98(5 Pt 1):853–860.

DiGiovanna JJ (2001). Isotretinoin effects on bone. *Journal of the American Academy of Dermatology* 45(5):S176–S182.

DiGiovanna JJ, Langman CB, Tschen EH (2004). Effect of a single course of isotretinoin therapy on bone mineral density in adolescent patients with severe, recalcitrant, nodular acne. *Journal of the American Academy of Dermatology* 51(5):709–717.

Dong D, Ruuska SE, Levinthal DJ, Noy N (1999). Distinct roles for cellular retinoic acid-binding proteins I and II in regulating signaling by retinoic acid. *Journal of Biological Chemistry* 274(34):23695–23698.

Dubertret L, Alirezai M, Rostain G, *et al*. (2003). The use of lymecycline in the treatment of moderate to severe acne vulgaris: a comparison of the efficacy and safety of two dosing regimens. *European Journal of Dermatology* 13(1):44–48.

Esterly NB, Furey NL, Flanagan LE (1978). The effect of antimicrobial agents on leukocyte chemotaxis. *Journal of Investigative Dermatology* 70(1):51–55.

Esterly NB, Koransky JS, Furey NL, Trevisan M (1984). Neutrophil chemotaxis in patients with acne receiving oral tetracycline therapy. *Archives of Dermatology* 120(10):1308–1313.

Fernandez-Obregon A C (2000). Azithromycin for the treatment of acne. *International Journal of Dermatology* 39(1):45–50.

Fitton A, Goa KL (1991). Azelaic acid. A review of its pharmacological properties and therapeutic efficacy in acne and hyperpigmentary skin disorders. *Drugs* 41(5):780–798.

Flynn WJ, Freeman PG, Wickboldt LG (1987). Pancreatitis associated with isotretinoin-induced hypertriglyceridemia. *Annals of Internal Medicine* 107(1):63.

Friedman DI (2005). Medication-induced intracranial hypertension in dermatology. *American Journal of Clinical Dermatology* **6**(1): 29–37.

Friedman GD, Ury HK (1980). Initial screening for carcinogenicity of commonly used drugs. *Journal of the National Cancer Institute* **65**(4):723–733.

Friedman SJ (1987). Leukopenia and neutropenia associated with isotretinoin therapy. *Archives of Dermatology* **123**(3):293–295.

Genvert GI, Cohen EJ, Donnenfeld ED, Blecher MH (1985). Erythema multiforme after use of topical sulfacetamide. *American Journal of Ophthalmology* **99**(4):465–468.

Godfrey KM, James MP (1990). Treatment of severe acne with isotretinoin in patients with inflammatory bowel disease. *British Journal of Dermatology* **123**(5):653–655.

Goltz RW, Coryell GM, Schnieders JR, Neidert GL (1985). A comparison of Cleocin T 1 percent solution and Cleocin T 1 percent lotion in the treatment of acne vulgaris. *Cutis* **36**(3):265–268.

Golub LM, Sorsa T, Lee HM (1995). Doxycycline inhibits neutrophil (PMN)-type matrix metalloproteinases in human adult periodontitis gingiva. *Journal of Clinical Periodontology* **22**(2):100–109.

Goodfellow A, Alaghband-Zadeh J, Carter G, et al. (1984). Oral spironolactone improves acne vulgaris and reduces sebum excretion. *British Journal of Dermatology* **111**(2):209–214.

Gottschalk HR, Stone OJ (1976). Stevens–Johnson syndrome from ophthalmic sulfonamide. *Archives of Dermatology* **112**(4):513–514.

Goulden V, Clark SM, McGeown C, Cunliffe WJ (1997). Treatment of acne with intermittent isotretinoin. *British Journal of Dermatology* **137**(1):106–108.

Groenendal H, Rampen FH (1990). Methotrexate and trimethoprim-sulphamethoxazole–a potentially hazardous combination. *Clinical and Experimental Dermatology* **15**(5):358–360.

Guerin C, Laterra J, Masnyk T, Golub LM, Brem H (1992). Selective endothelial growth inhibition by tetracyclines that inhibit collagenase. *Biochemical and Biophysical Research Communications* **188**(2):740–745.

Gupta AK, Nicol K (2004). The use of sulfur in dermatology. *Journal of Drugs in Dermatology* **3**(4):427–431.

Halpagi P, Grigg J, Klistorner A, Damian DL (2008). Night blindness following low-dose isotretinoin. *Journal of the European Academy of Dermatology and Venereology* **22**(7):893–894.

Healy DP, Dansereau RJ, Dunn AB, Clendening CE, Mounts AW, Deepe GS Jr (1997). Reduced tetracycline bioavailability caused by magnesium aluminum silicate in liquid formulations of bismuth subsalicylate. *Annals of Pharmacotherapy* **31**(12):1460–1464.

Helms SE, Bredle DL, Zajic J, Jarjoura D, Brodell RT, Krishnarao I (1997). Oral contraceptive failure rates and oral antibiotics. *Journal of the American Academy of Dermatology* **36**(5 Pt 1):705–710.

Huang C, Ma WY, Dawson MI, Rincon M, Flavell RA, Dong Z (1997). Blocking activator protein-1 activity, but not activating retinoic acid response element, is required for the antitumor promotion effect of retinoic acid. *Proceedings of the National Academy of Sciences of the United States of America* **94**(11):5826–5830.

Hull PR, D'Arcy C (2005). Acne, depression, and suicide. *Dermatologic Clinics* **23**(4):665–674.

Igarashi K, Ishitsuka H, Kaji A (1969). Comparative studies on the mechanism of action of lincomycin, streptomycin, and erythromycin. *Biochemical and Biophysical Research Communications* **37**(3):499–504.

Jick H, Derby LE (1995). A large population-based follow-up study of trimethoprim-sulfamethoxazole, trimethoprim, and cephalexin for uncommon serious drug toxicity. *Pharmacotherapy* **15**(4):428–432.

Jick H, Jick SS, Gurewich V, Myers MW, Vasilakis C (1995). Risk of idiopathic cardiovascular death and nonfatal venous thromboembolism in women using oral contraceptives with differing progestagen components. *Lancet* **346**(8990):1589–1593.

Jick SS, Kremers HM, Vasilakis-Scaramozza C (2000). Isotretinoin use and risk of depression, psychotic symptoms, suicide, and attempted suicide. *Archives of Dermatology* **136**(10):1231–1236.

Jick SS, Kaye JA, Russmann S, Jick H (2006). Risk of nonfatal venous thromboembolism with oral contraceptives containing norgestimate or desogestrel compared with oral contraceptives containing levonorgestrel. *Contraception* **73**(6):566–570.

Jorro G, Morales C, Braso JV, Pelaez A (1996). Anaphylaxis to erythromycin. *Annals of Allergy, Asthma, and Immunology* **77**(6):456–458.

Kaymak Y, Ilter N (2006). The effectiveness of intermittent isotretinoin treatment in mild or moderate acne. *Journal of the European Academy of Dermatology and Venereology* **20**(10):1256–1260.

Keeffe EB, Reis TC, Berland JE (1982). Hepatotoxicity to both erythromycin estolate and erythromycin ethylsuccinate. *Digestive Diseases and Sciences* **27**(8):701–704.

Kloppenburg M, Verweij CL, Miltenburg AM, et al. (1995). The influence of tetracyclines on T cell activation. *Clinical and Experimental Immunology* **102**(3):635–641.

Kus S, Yucelten D, Aytug A (2005). Comparison of efficacy of azithromycin vs. doxycycline in the treatment of acne vulgaris. *Clinical and Experimental Dermatology* **30**(3):215–220.

Lammer EJ, Chen DT, Hoar RM, et al. (1985). Retinoic acid embryopathy. *New England Journal of Medicine* **313**(14):837–841.

Latriano L, Tzimas G, Wong F, Wills RJ (1997). The percutaneous absorption of topically applied tretinoin and its effect on endogenous concentrations of tretinoin and its metabolites after single doses or long-term use. *Journal of the American Academy of Dermatology* **36**(3 Pt 2):S37–S46.

Lavker RM, Leyden JJ, Thorne EG (1992). An ultrastructural study of the effects of topical tretinoin on microcomedones. *Clinical Therapeutics* **14**(6):773–780.

Lawrenson RA, Seaman HE, Sundstrom A, Williams TJ, Farmer RD (2000). Liver damage associated with minocycline use in acne: a systematic review of the published literature and pharmacovigilance data. *Drug Safety* **23**(4):333–349.

Layton AM, Hughes BR, Hull SM, Eady EA, Cunliffe WJ (1992). Seborrhoea–an indicator for poor clinical response in acne patients treated with antibiotics. *Clinical and Experimental Dermatology* **17**(3):173–175.

Lee AG (1995). Pseudotumor cerebri after treatment with tetracycline and isotretinoin for acne. *Cutis* **55**(3):165–168.

Lee WL, Shalita AR, Suntharalingam K, Fikrig SM (1982). Neutrophil chemotaxis by *Propionibacterium acnes* lipase and its inhibition. *Infection and Immunity* **35**(1):71–78.

Lehucher Ceyrac D, Chaspoux C, Sulimovic L, Morel P, Lefrencq H (1998) Aggravation of acne by isotretinoin. 6 case, predictive factors. *Annals of Dermatology and Venereology* **125**(8):496–499

Lewis MA, Heinemann LA, Spitzer WO, MacRae KD, Bruppacher R (1997). The use of oral contraceptives and the occurrence of acute myocardial infarction in young women. Results from the Transnational Study on Oral Contraceptives and the Health of Young Women. *Contraception* **56**(3):129–140.

Lewis PA, Kearney PJ (1997). Pseudotumor cerebri induced by minocycline treatment for acne vulgaris. *Acta Dermato-Venereologica* **77**(1):83.

Leyden JJ, Hickman JG, Jarratt MT, Stewart DM, Levy SF (2001a). The efficacy and safety of a combination benzoyl peroxide/clindamycin topical gel compared with benzoyl peroxide alone and a benzoyl peroxide/erythromycin combination product. *Journal of Cutaneous Medicine and Surgery* **5**(1):37–42.

Leyden JJ, Berger RS, Dunlap FE, Ellis CN, Connolly MA, Levy SF (2001b). Comparison of the efficacy and safety of a combination topical gel formulation of benzoyl peroxide and clindamycin with benzoyl peroxide, clindamycin and vehicle gel in the treatments of acne vulgaris. *American Journal of Clinical Dermatology* **2**(1):33–39.

Leyden J, Lowe N, Kakita L, Draelos Z (2001c). Comparison of treatment of acne vulgaris with alternate-day applications of tazarotene 0.1% gel and once-daily applications of adapalene 0.1% gel: a randomized trial. *Cutis* **67**(6 Suppl):10–16.

Lin AN, Reimer RJ, Carter DM (1988). Sulfur revisited. *Journal of the American Academy of Dermatology* 18(3):553–558

[Ling TC, Parkin G, Islam J, Seukeran DC, Cunliffe WJ (2001). What is the cumulative effect of long-term, low-dose isotretinoin on the development of DISH? *British Journal of Dermatology* 144(3):630–632.

Liu PT, Krutzik SR, Kim J, Modlin RL (2005). Cutting edge: all-trans retinoic acid down-regulates TLR2 expression and function. *Journal of Immunology* 174(5):2467–2470.

Lookingbill DP, Chalker DK, Lindholm JS, *et al.* (1997). Treatment of acne with a combination clindamycin/benzoyl peroxide gel compared with clindamycin gel, benzoyl peroxide gel and vehicle gel: combined results of two double-blind investigations. *Journal of the American Academy of Dermatology* 37(4):590–595.

Loube SD, Quirk RA (1975). Letter: Breast cancer associated with administration of spironolactone. *Lancet* 1(7922):1428–1429.

Maheshwai N (2007). Are young infants treated with erythromycin at risk for developing hypertrophic pyloric stenosis? *Archives of Disease in Childhood* 92(3):271–273.

Mangelsdorf DJ, Ong ES, Dyck JA, Evans RM (1990). Nuclear receptor that identifies a novel retinoic acid response pathway. *Nature* 345(6272):224–229.

Marcelo CL, Madison KC (1984). Regulation of the expression of epidermal keratinocyte proliferation and differentiation by vitamin A analogs. *Archives of Dermatological Research* 276(6):381–389.

Margolis DJ, Hoffstad O, Bilker W (2007). Association or lack of association between tetracycline class antibiotics used for acne vulgaris and lupus erythematosus. *British Journal of Dermatology* 157:540–546.

Marqueling AL, Zane LT (2007). Depression and suicidal behavior in acne patients treated with isotretinoin: a systematic review. *Seminars in Cutaneous Medicine and Surgery* 26(4):210–220.

Martin B, Meunier C, Montels D, Watts O (1998). Chemical stability of adapalene and tretinoin when combined with benzoyl peroxide in presence and in absence of visible light and ultraviolet radiation. *British Journal of Dermatology* 139(52 Suppl):8–11.

Mayer-da-Silva A, Gollnick H, Detmar M, *et al.* (1989). Effects of azelaic acid on sebaceous gland, sebum excretion rate and keratinization pattern in human skin. An *in vivo* and *in vitro* study. *Acta Dermato-Venereologica Supplementum* 143:20–30.

McGhan LJ, Merchant SN (2003). Erythromycin ototoxicity. *Otology and Neurotology* 24(4):701–702.

McCarter TL, Chen YK (1992). Marked hyperlipidemia and pancreatitis associated with isotretinoin therapy. *American Journal of Gastroenterology* 87(12):1855–1858.

Menter A (2000). Pharmacokinetics and safety of tazarotene. *Journal of the American Academy of Dermatology* 43(2 Pt 3):S31–35.

Mills OH Jr, Kligman AM (1983). Assay of comedolytic activity in acne patients. *Acta Dermato-Venereologica* 63(1):68–71.

Milstone EB, McDonald AJ, Scholhamer CF Jr (1981). Pseudomembranous colitis after topical application of clindamycin. *Archives of Dermatology* 117(3):154–155.

Monzon RI, LaPres JJ, Hudson LG (1996). Regulation of involucrin gene expression by retinoic acid and glucocorticoids. *Cell Growth and Differentiation* 7(12):1751–1759.

Morelli R, Lanzarini M, Vincenzi C, Reggiani M (1989). Contact dermatitis due to benzoyl peroxide. *Contact Dermatitis* 20(3):238–239.

Mouton RW, Jordaan HF, Schneider JW (2004). A new type of minocycline-induced cutaneous hyperpigmentation. *Clinical and Experimental Dermatology* 29(1):8–14.

Mylonakis E, Ryan ET, Calderwood SB (2001). *Clostridium difficile*-associated diarrhea: a review. *Archives of Internal Medicine* 161(4):525–533.

Nelson AM, Gilliland KL, Cong Z, Thiboutot DM (2006). 13-cis Retinoic acid induces apoptosis and cell cycle arrest in human SEB-1 sebocytes. *Journal of Investigative Dermatology* 126(10):2178–2189.

Neu HC (1991). Clinical microbiology of azithromycin. *American Journal of Medicine* 91(3A):12S–18S.

Neuvonen PJ (1976). Interactions with the absorption of tetracyclines. *Drugs* 11(1):45–54.

Nishimura G, Mugishima H, Hirao J, Yamato M (1997). Generalized metaphyseal modification with cone-shaped epiphyses following long-term administration of 13-cis-retinoic acid. *European Journal of Pediatrics* 156(6):432–435.

Nyirady J, Lucas C, Yusuf M, Mignone P, Wisniewski S (2002). The stability of tretinoin in tretinoin gel microsphere 0.1%. *Cutis* 70(5):295–298.

Oertel YC (2007). Black thyroid syndrome. *Thyroid* 17(9):905.

Overdiek HW, Hermens WA, Merkus FW (1985). New insights into the pharmacokinetics of spironolactone. *Clinical Pharmacology and Therapeutics* 38(4):469–474.

Overdiek HW, Merkus FW (1986). Influence of food on the bioavailability of spironolactone. *Clinical Pharmacology and Therapeutics* 40(5):531–536.

Ozdemir MA, Kose M, Karakukcu M, Ferahbas A, Patiroglu T, Koklu E (2007). Isotretinoin-induced agranulocytosis. *Pediatric Dermatology* 24(4):425–426.

Parker F (1987). A comparison of clindamycin 1% solution versus clindamycin 1% gel in the treatment of acne vulgaris. *International Journal of Dermatology* 26(2):121–122.

Parry MF, Rha CK (1986). Pseudomembranous colitis caused by topical clindamycin phosphate. *Archives of Dermatology* 122(5):583–584.

Parsad D, Pandhi R, Nagpal R, Negi KS (2001). Azithromycin monthly pulse *vs.* daily doxycycline in the treatment of acne vulgaris. *Journal of Dermatology* 28(1):1–4.

Pelletier F, Puzenat E, Blanc D, Faivre B, Humbert P, Aubin F (2003). Minocycline-induced cutaneous polyarteritis nodosa with antineutrophil cytoplasmic antibodies. *European Journal of Dermatology* 13(4):396–398.

Petkovich M, Brand N J, Krust A, Chambon P (1987). A human retinoic acid receptor which belongs to the family of nuclear receptors. *Nature* 330(6147):444–450.

Phelps DL, Karim Z (1977). Spironolactone: relationship between concentrations of dethioacetylated metabolite in human serum and milk. *Journal of Pharmaceutical Sciences* 66(8):1203.

Phillips ME, Eastwood JB, Curtis JR, Gower PC, De Wardener HE (1974). Tetracycline poisoning in renal failure. *British Medical Journal* 2(5911):149–151.

Pisciotta AV (1993). Agranulocytosis during antibiotic therapy: drug sensitivity or sepsis? *American Journal of Hematology* 42(1):132–137.

Presland RB, Tomic-Canic M, Lewis SP, Dale BA (2001). Regulation of human profilaggrin promoter activity in cultured epithelial cells by retinoic acid and glucocorticoids. *Journal of Dermatological Science* 27(3):192–205.

Rafiei R, Yaghoobi R (2006). Azithromycin versus tetracycline in the treatment of acne vulgaris. *Journal of Dermatological Treatment* 17(4):217–221.

Reddy D, Siegel CA, Sands BE, Kane S (2006). Possible association between isotretinoin and inflammatory bowel disease. *American Journal of Gastroenterology* 101(7):1569–1573.

Robins EJ, Breathnach AS, Bennett D, *et al.* (1985). Ultrastructural observations on the effect of azelaic acid on normal human melanocytes and a human melanoma cell line in tissue culture. *British Journal of Dermatology* 113(6):687–697.

Roytman M, Frumkin A, Bohn TG (1988). Pseudotumor cerebri caused by isotretinoin. *Cutis* 42(5):399–400.

Rubin Z (1977). Ophthalmic sulfonamide-induced Stevens–Johnson syndrome. *Archives of Dermatology* 113(2):235–236.

Sadick NS (2007). Systemic antibacterial agents. In: Wolverton SE (ed). *Comprehensive Dermatologic Drug Therapy*, 2nd edn. WB Saunders, Philadelphia, ch 3, p. 28.

Sainte-Marie I, Tenaud I, Jumbou O, Dreno B (1999). Minocycline modulation of alpha-MSH production by keratinocytes *in vitro*. *Acta Dermato-Venereologica* 79(4):265–267.

Sapadin AN, Fleischmajer R (2006). Tetracyclines: nonantibiotic properties and their clinical implications. *Journal of the American Academy of Dermatology* 54:258–265.

Schaffer JV, Davidson DM, McNiff JM, Bolognia JL (2001). Perinuclear antineutrophilic cytoplasmic antibody-positive cutaneous polyarteritis nodosa associated with minocycline therapy for acne vulgaris. *Journal of the American Academy of Dermatology* 44(2):198–206.

Scheinman PL, Peck GL, Rubinow DR, DiGiovanna JJ, Abangan DL, Ravin PD (1990). Acute depression from isotretinoin. *Journal of the American Academy of Dermatology* 22(6 Pt 1):1112–1114.

Schmidt JB, Knobler R, Neumann R, Poitschek C (1983). [External erythromycin therapy of acne]. *Zeitschrift für Hautkrankheiten* 58(24):1754–1760.

Seukeran DC, Cunliffe WJ (1999). The treatment of acne fulminans: a review of 25 cases. *British Journal of Dermatology* 141(2):307–309.

Shalita AR (1987). Mucocutaneous and systemic toxicity of retinoids: monitoring and management. *Dermatologica* 175(1 Suppl):151–157.

Shapiro LE, Knowles SR, Shear NH (1997). Comparative safety of tetracycline, minocycline, and doxycycline. *Archives of Dermatology* 133(10):1224–1230.

Shapiro S, Szarewski A (2007). Oral contraceptives, menopausal treatment, and cancer. *Lancet Oncology* 8(10):867.

Shaw JC (2000). Low-dose adjunctive spironolactone in the treatment of acne in women: a retrospective analysis of 85 consecutively treated patients. *Journal of the American Academy of Dermatology* 43(3):498–502.

Shaw JC, White LE (2002). Long-term safety of spironolactone in acne: results of an 8-year followup study. *Journal of Cutaneous Medicine and Surgery* 6(6):541–545.

Shroot B (1998). Pharmacodynamics and pharmacokinetics of topical adapalene. *Journal of the American Academy of Dermatology* 39(2 Pt 3):S17–S24.

Simonart T, Dramaix M (2005). Treatment of acne with topical antibiotics: lessons from clinical studies. *British Journal of Dermatology* 153(2):395–403.

Skidmore R, Kovach R, Walker C, *et al.* (2003). Effects of subantimicrobial-dose doxycycline in the treatment of moderate acne. *Archives of Dermatology* 139(4):459–464.

Skov MJ, Quigley JW, Bucks DA (1997). Topical delivery system for tretinoin: research and clinical implications. *Journal of Pharmaceutical Sciences* 86(10):1138–1143.

Smith K, Leyden JJ (2005). Safety of doxycycline and minocycline: a systematic review. *Clinical Therapeutics* 27(9):1329–1342.

Stern RS, Rosa F, Baum C (1984). Isotretinoin and pregnancy. *Journal of the American Academy of Dermatology* 10(5 Pt 1):851–854.

Stewart DM, Torok HM, Weiss JS, Plott RT (2006). Dose-ranging efficacy of new once-daily extended-release minocycline for acne vulgaris. *Cutis* 78(4 Suppl):11–20.

Stoughton RB, Cornell RC, Gange RW, Walter JF (1980). Double-blind comparison of topical 1 percent clindamycin phosphate (Cleocin T) and oral tetracycline 500 mg/day in the treatment of acne vulgaris. *Cutis* 26(4):424–425, 429.

Swinyer LJ, Baker MD, Swinyer TA, Mills OH Jr (1988). A comparative study of benzoyl peroxide and clindamycin phosphate for treating acne vulgaris. *British Journal of Dermatology* 119(5):615–622.

Szarewski A (2005). Oral oestrogen–progestagen contraceptives, menopausal treatment, and cancer. *Lancet Oncology* 6(10):736–737.

Tamargo RJ, Bok RA, Brem H (1991). Angiogenesis inhibition by minocycline. *Cancer Research* 51(2):672–675.

Tang-Liu DD, Matsumoto RM, Usansky JI (1999). Clinical pharmacokinetics and drug metabolism of tazarotene: a novel topical treatment for acne and psoriasis. *Clinical Pharmacokinetics* 37(4):273–287.

Tauber U, Weiss C, Matthes H (1992). Percutaneous absorption of azelaic acid in humans. *Experimental Dermatology* 1(4):176–179.

Tenaud I, Khammari A, Dreno B (2007). *In vitro* modulation of TLR-2, CD1d and IL-10 by adapalene on normal human skin and acne inflammatory lesions. *Experimental Dermatology* 16(6):500–506.

Thomas DR, Dover JS, Camp RD (1987). Pancytopenia induced by the interaction between methotrexate and trimethoprim–sulfamethoxazole. *Journal of the American Academy of Dermatology* 17(6):1055–1056.

Thomsen RJ, Stranieri A, Knutson D, Strauss JS (1980). Topical clindamycin treatment of acne. Clinical, surface lipid composition, and quantitative surface microbiology response. *Archives of Dermatology* 116(9):1031–1034.

Tsukada M, Schroder M, Roos TC, *et al.* (2000). 13-cis Retinoic acid exerts its specific activity on human sebocytes through selective intracellular isomerization to all-trans retinoic acid and binding to retinoid acid receptors. *Journal of Investigative Dermatology* 115(2):321–327.

Uchida G, Yoshimura K, Kitano Y, Okazaki M, Harii K (2003). Tretinoin reverses upregulation of matrix metalloproteinase-13 in human keloid-derived fibroblasts. *Experimental Dermatology* 12 (2 Suppl):35–42.

Waisman M (1988). Agranulocytosis from isotretinoin. *Journal of the American Academy of Dermatology* 18(2 Pt 1):395–396.

Waller JM, Dreher F, Behnam S, *et al.* (2006). 'Keratolytic' properties of benzoyl peroxide and retinoic acid resemble salicylic acid in man. *Skin Pharmacology and Physiology* 19(5):283–289.

Weinstein GD, Krueger GG, Lowe NJ, *et al.* (1997). Tazarotene gel, a new retinoid, for topical therapy of psoriasis: vehicle-controlled study of safety, efficacy, and duration of therapeutic effect. *Journal of the American Academy of Dermatology* 37(1):85–92.

Wennberg RP, Ahlfors CE (2006). A different view on bilirubin binding. *Pediatrics* 118(2):846–847.

Wiegratz I, Jung-Hoffmann C, Kuhl H (1995). Effect of two oral contraceptives containing ethinylestradiol and gestodene or norgestimate upon androgen parameters and serum binding proteins. *Contraception* 51(6):341–346.

Yao JS, Chen Y, Zhai W, Xu K, Young WL, Yang GY (2004). Minocycline exerts multiple inhibitory effects on vascular endothelial growth factor-induced smooth muscle cell migration: the role of ERK1/2, PI3K, and matrix metalloproteinases. *Circulation Research* 95(4):364–371.

Yao JS, Shen F, Young WL, Yang GY (2007). Comparison of doxycycline and minocycline in the inhibition of VEGF-induced smooth muscle cell migration. *Neurochemistry International* 50(3):524–530.

Yemisci A, Gorgulu A, Piskin S (2005). Effects and side-effects of spironolactone therapy in women with acne. *Journal of the European Academy of Dermatology and Venereology* 19(2):163–166.

Yu Z, Sefton J, Lew-Kaya D, Walker P, Yu D, Tang-Liu DD (2003). Pharmacokinetics of tazarotene cream 0.1% after a single dose and after repeat topical applications at clinical or exaggerated application rates in patients with acne vulgaris or photodamaged skin. *Clinical Pharmacokinetics* 42(10):921–929.

Zachariae H (1988). Delayed wound healing and keloid formation following argon laser treatment or dermabrasion during isotretinoin treatment. *British Journal of Dermatology* 118(5):703–706.

Zane LT, Leyden WA, Marqueling AL, Manos MM (2006). A population-based analysis of laboratory abnormalities during isotretinoin therapy for acne vulgaris. *Archives of Dermatology* **142**(8):1016–1022.

Chapter 3

Alexiades-Armenakas M (2006). Long-pulsed dye laser-mediated photodynamic therapy combined with topical therapy for mild to severe comedonal, inflammatory, or cystic acne. *Journal of Drugs in Dermatology* **5**(1):45–55.

Arakane K, Ryu A, Hayashi C, *et al.* (1996). Singlet oxygen (1 delta g) generation from coproporphyrin in *Propionibacterium acnes* on irradiation. *Biochemical and Biophysical Research Communications* **223**(3): 578–582.

Ashkenazi H, Malik Z, Harth Y, Nitzan Y (2003). Eradication of *Propionibacterium acnes* by its endogenic porphyrins after illumination with high intensity blue light. *FEMS Immunology and Medical Microbiology* **35**(1):17–24.

Barnard JA, Bascom CC, Lyons RM, Sipes NJ, Moses HL (1988) Transforming growth factor beta in the control of epidermal proliferation. *American Journal of Medical Sciences* **296**(3):159–163.

Bogle MA, Dover JS, Arndt KA, Mordon S (2007). Evaluation of the 1,540 nm erbium:glass laser in the treatment of inflammatory facial acne. *Dermatologic Surgery* **33**(7):810–817.

Choi YS, Suh HS, Yoon MY, Min SU, Lee DH, Suh DH (2010) Intense pulsed light *vs.* pulsed-dye laser in the treatment of facial acne: a randomized split-face trial. *Journal of the European Academy of Dermatology and Venereology* **24**(7):773–780.

Clayton TH, Stables GI (2005) Reactivation of ophthalmic herpes zoster following pulsed-dye laser treatment for inflammatory acne vulgaris. *British Journal of Dermatology* **152**(3):569–570.

Dahan S, Lagarde JM, Turlier V, Courrech L, Mordon S (2004). Treatment of neck lines and forehead rhytids with a nonablative 1540 nm Er:glass laser: a controlled clinical study combined with the measurement of the thickness and the mechanical properties of the skin. *Dermatologic Surgery* **30**(6):872–879.

Divaris DX, Kennedy JC, Pottier RH (1990). Phototoxic damage to sebaceous glands and hair follicles of mice after systemic administration of 5-aminolevulinic acid correlates with localized protoporphyrin IX fluorescence. *American Journal of Pathology* **136**(4):891–897.

Fournier N, Mordon S (2005). Nonablative remodeling with a 1,540 nm erbium:glass laser. *Dermatologic Surgery* **31**:1227–1236.

Fritsch C, Goerz G, Ruzicka T (1998). Photodynamic therapy in dermatology. *Archives of Dermatology* **134**(2):207–214.

Goldberg DJ, Russell BA (2006). Combination blue (415 nm) and red (633 nm) LED phototherapy in the treatment of mild to severe acne vulgaris. *Journal of Cosmetic and Laser Therapy* **8**(2):71–75.

Goldman MP, Boyce SM (2003). A single-center study of aminolevulinic acid and 417 nm photodynamic therapy in the treatment of moderate to severe acne vulgaris. *Journal of Drugs in Dermatology* **2**(4):393–396.

Hongcharu W, Taylor CR, Chang Y, Aghassi D, Suthamjariya K, Anderson RR (2000). Topical ALA-photodynamic therapy for the treatment of acne vulgaris. *Journal of Investigative Dermatology* **115**(2):183–192.

Hörfelt C, Funk J, Frohm-Nilsson M, Wiegleb Edström D, Wennberg AM (2006). Topical methyl aminolaevulinate photodynamic therapy for treatment of facial acne vulgaris: results of a randomized, controlled study. *British Journal of Dermatology* **155**(3):608–613.

Jih MH, Friedman PM, Goldberg LH, Robles M, Glaich AS, Kimyai-Asadi A (2006). The 1450 nm diode laser for facial inflammatory acne vulgaris: dose-response and 12-month follow-up study. *Journal of the American Academy of Dermatology* **55**(1):80–87.

Jope EM, O'Brien JRP (1945). Spectral absorption and fluorescence of coproporphyrin isomers I and III and the melting-points of their methyl esters. *Biochemical Journal* **39**(3):239–244.

Karsai S, Schmitt L, Raulin C (2010) The pulsed-dye laser as an adjuvant treatment modality in acne vulgaris: a randomized controlled single-blinded trial. *British Journal of Dermatology* **163**(2):395–401.

Kawada A, Aragane Y, Kameyama H, Sangen Y, Tezuka T (2002). Acne phototherapy with a high-intensity, enhanced, narrow-band, blue light source: an open study and *in vitro* investigation. *Journal of Dermatological Science* **30**(2):129–135.

Kelly KM, Nelson JS, Lask GP, Geronemus RG, Bernstein LJ (1999). Cryogen spray cooling in combination with nonablative laser treatment of facial rhytides. *Archives of Dermatology* **135**:691–694.

Kennedy JC, Pottier RH, Pross DC (1990). Photodynamic therapy with endogenous protoporphyrin IX: basic principles and present clinical experience. *Journal of Photochemistry and Photobiology B: Biology* **6**(1–2):143–148.

Lee WL, Shalita AR, Poh-Fitzpatrick MB (1978). Comparative studies of porphyrin production in *Propionibacterium acnes* and *Propionibacterium granulosum*. *Journal of Bacteriology* **133**(2):811–815.

Leheta TM (2009) Role of the 585-nm pulsed-dye laser in the treatment of acne in comparison with other topical therapeutic modalities. *Journal of Cosmetic and Laser Therapy* **11**(2):118–124.

Lim W, Lee S, Kim I, *et al.* (2007). The anti-inflammatory mechanism of 635 nm light-emitting-diode irradiation compared with existing COX inhibitors. *Lasers in Surgery and Medicine* **39**(7):614–621.

Lupton JR, Alster TS (2001). Nonablative cutaneous laser resurfacing using a 1.54 μm erbium-doped phosphate glass laser: a clinical and histologic study. *Lasers in Surgery and Medicine* **13**:S46.

McDaniel DH, Geronemus RG, Weiss RA, Weiss M (2007). LED photomodulation for acne. *Lasers in Surgery and Medicine* **39**(19 Suppl):27.

[Mordon S, Capon A, Creusy C, *et al.* (2000). *In vivo* experimental evaluation of skin remodeling by using an Er:Glass laser with contact cooling. *Lasers in Surgery and Medicine* **27**:1–9.

Morton CA, Scholefield RD, Whitehurst C, Birch J (2005). An open study to determine the efficacy of blue light in the treatment of mild to moderate acne. *Journal of Dermatological Treatment* **16**(4):219–223.

Nestor MS, Gold MH, Kauvar AN, *et al.* (2006). The use of photodynamic therapy in dermatology: results of a consensus conference. *Journal of Drugs in Dermatology* **5**(2):140–154.

Orringer JS, Kang S, Hamilton T, *et al.* (2004) Treatment of acne vulgaris with a pulsed-dye laser: a randomized controlled trial. *Journal of the American Medical Association* **291**(23):2834–2839.

Orringer JS, Kang S, Maier L, *et al.* (2007). A randomized, controlled, split-face clinical trial of 1320 nm Nd:YAG laser therapy in the treatment of acne vulgaris. *Journal of the American Academy of Dermatology* **56**(3):432–438.

Paithankar DY, Ross EV, Saleh BA, Blair MA, Graham BS (2002). Acne treatment with a 1,450 nm wavelength laser and cryogen spray cooling. *Lasers in Surgery and Medicine* **31**(2):106–114.

Papageorgiou P, Katsambas A, Chu A (2000). Phototherapy with blue (415 nm) and red (660 nm) light in the treatment of acne vulgaris. *British Journal of Dermatology* **142**(5):973–978.

[Perez-Maldonado A, Runger TM, Krejci-Papa N (2007). The 1,450 nm diode laser reduces sebum production in facial skin: a possible mode of action of its effectiveness for the treatment of acne vulgaris. *Lasers in Surgery and Medicine* **39**(2):189–192.

Pollock B, Turner D, Stringer MR (2004). Topical aminolaevulinic acid-photodynamic therapy for the treatment of acne vulgaris: a study of clinical efficacy and mechanism of action. *British Journal of Dermatology* **151**(3):616–622.

Prieto VG, Zhang PS, Sadick NS (2005). Evaluation of pulsed light and radiofrequency combined for the treatment of acne vulgaris with histologic analysis of facial skin biopsies. *Journal of Cosmetic and Laser Therapy* **7**(2):63–68.

Ruiz-Esparza J, Gomez JB (2003). Nonablative radiofrequency for active acne vulgaris: the use of deep dermal heat in the treatment of moderate to severe acne vulgaris (thermotherapy): a report of 22 patients. *Dermatologic Surgery* 29(4):333–339.

Ruiz-Rodriguez R, Lopez L, Candelas D, Zelickson B (2007). Enhanced efficacy of photodynamic therapy after fractional resurfacing: fractional photodynamic rejuvenation. *Journal of Drugs in Dermatology* 6(8):818–820.

Santos MA, Belo VG, Santos G (2005). Effectiveness of photodynamic therapy with topical 5-aminolevulinic acid and intense pulsed light versus intense pulsed light alone in the treatment of acne vulgaris: comparative study. *Dermatologic Surgery* 31(8 Pt 1):910–915.

Seaton ED, Charakida A, Mouser PE, Grace I, Clement RM, Chu AC (2003). Pulsed-dye laser treatment for inflammatory acne vulgaris: randomised controlled trial. *Lancet* 362(9393):1347–1352.

Seaton ED, Mouser PE, Charakida A, Alam S, Seldon PM, Chu AC (2006). Investigation of the mechanism of action of nonablative pulsed-dye laser therapy in photorejuvenation and inflammatory acne vulgaris. *British Journal of Dermatology* 155(4):748–755.

Shnitkind E, Yaping E, Geen S, Shalita AR, Lee WL (2006). Anti-inflammatory properties of narrow-band blue light. *Journal of Drugs in Dermatology* 5(7):605–610.

Sigurdsson V, Knulst AC, van Weelden H (1997). Phototherapy of acne vulgaris with visible light. *Dermatology* 194(3):256–260.

Taub AF (2004). Photodynamic therapy for the treatment of acne: a pilot study. *Journal of Drugs in Dermatology* 3(6 Suppl):S10–S14.

Uebelhoer NS, Bogle MA, Dover JS, Arndt KA, Rohrer TE (2007). Comparison of stacked pulses versus double-pass treatments of facial acne with a 1,450 nm laser. *Dermatologic Surgery* 33(5):552–559.

Wahl SM, Swisher J, McCartney-Francis N, Chen W (2004). TGF-beta: the perpetrator of immune suppression by regulatory T cells and suicidal T cells. *Journal of Leukocyte Biology* 76(1):15–24.

Wang SQ, Counters JT, Flor ME, Zelickson BD (2006). Treatment of inflammatory facial acne with the 1,450 nm diode laser alone versus microdermabrasion plus the 1,450 nm laser: a randomized, split-face trial. *Dermatologic Surgery* 32(2):249–255.

Wiegell SR, Wulf HC (2006a). Photodynamic therapy of acne vulgaris using methyl aminolaevulinate: a blinded, randomized, controlled trial. *British Journal of Dermatology* 154(5):969–976.

Wiegell SR, Wulf HC (2006b). Photodynamic therapy of acne vulgaris using 5-aminolevulinic acid versus methyl aminolevulinate. *Journal of the American Academy of Dermatology* 54(4):647–651.

Chapter 4

Abergel RP, Pizzurro D, Meeker CA, *et al.* (1985). Biochemical composition of the connective tissue in keloids and analysis of collagen metabolism in keloid fibroblast cultures. *Journal of Investigative Dermatology* 84(5):384–390.

Alam M, Omura N, Kaminer MS (2005). Subcision for acne scarring: technique and outcomes in 40 patients. *Dermatologic Surgery* 31(3):310–317.

Alster TS (1994). Improvement of erythematous and hypertrophic scars by the 585-nm flashlamp-pumped pulsed dye laser. *Annals of Plastic Surgery* 32(2):186–190.

Alster TS, West TB (1996). Resurfacing of atrophic facial acne scars with a high-energy, pulsed carbon dioxide laser. *Dermatologic Surgery* 22(2):151–154.

Alster TS, Tanzi EL, Lazarus M (2007). The use of fractional laser photothermolysis for the treatment of atrophic scars. *Dermatologic Surgery* 33(3):295–299.

Aust MC, Fernandes D, Kolokythas P, Kaplan HM, Vogt PM (2008). Percutaneous collagen induction therapy: an alternative treatment for scars, wrinkles, and skin laxity. *Plastic and Reconstructive Surgery* 121(4):1421–1429.

Barnett JG, Barnett CR (2005). Treatment of acne scars with liquid silicone injections: 30-year perspective. *Dermatologic Surgery* 31(11 Pt 2):1542–1549.

Beer K (2007). A single-center, open-label study on the use of injectable poly-L-lactic acid for the treatment of moderate to severe scarring from acne or varicella. *Dermatologic Surgery* 33(2 Suppl):S159–S167.

Bernstein LJ, Kauvar AN, Grossman MC, Geronemus RG (1997). The short- and long-term side effects of carbon dioxide laser resurfacing. *Dermatologic Surgery* 23:519–525.

Botwood N, Lewanski C, Lowdell C (1999). The risks of treating keloids with radiotherapy. *British Journal of Radiology* 72(864):1222–1224.

Bogle MA, Arndt KA, Dover JS (2007). Plasma skin regeneration technology. *Journal of Drugs in Dermatology* 6(11):1110–1112.

Brodland DG, Cullimore KC, Roenigk RK, Gibson LE (1989). Depths of chemexfoliation induced by various concentrations and application techniques of trichloroacetic acid in a porcine model. *Journal of Dermatologic Surgery and Oncology* 15(9):967–971.

Brody HJ (1989). Variations and comparisons in medium-depth chemical peeling. *Journal of Dermatologic Surgery and Oncology* 15(9):953–963.

Butler PE, Gonzalez S, Randolph MA, Kim J, Kollias N, Yaremchuk MJ (2001). Quantitative and qualitative effects of chemical peeling on photo-aged skin: an experimental study. *Plastic and Reconstructive Surgery* 107(1):222–228.

Carroll LA, Hanasono MM, Mikulec AA, Kita M, Koch RJ (2002). Triamcinolone stimulates bFGF production and inhibits TGF-beta1 production by human dermal fibroblasts. *Dermatologic Surgery* 28(8):704–709.

Chan HHL, Manstein D, Yu CS, Shek S, Kono T, Wei WI (2007). The prevalence and risk factors of post-inflammatory hyperpigmentation after fractional resurfacing in Asians. *Lasers in Surgery and Medicine* 39:381–385.

Chapas AM, Brightman L, Sukal S, *et al.* (2008). Successful treatment of acneiform scarring with CO_2 ablative fractional resurfacing. *Lasers in Surgery and Medicine* 40(6):381–386.

Cho SB, Park CO, Chung WG, Lee KH, Lee JB, Chung KY (2006). Histometric and histochemical analysis of the effect of trichloroacetic acid concentration in the chemical reconstruction of skin scars method. *Dermatologic Surgery* 32(10):1231–1236.

Coleman SR (2006). Structural fat grafting: more than a permanent filler. *Plastic and Reconstructive Surgery* 118(3 Suppl):108S–120S.

Conn H, Nanda VS (2000). Prophylactic fluconazole promotes re-epithelialization in full-face carbon dioxide laser skin resurfacing. *Lasers in Surgery and Medicine* 26:201–207.

Dailey RA, Gray JF, Rubin MG, *et al.* (1998). Histopathologic changes of the eyelid skin following trichloroacetic acid chemical peel. *Ophthalmic Plastic and Reconstructive Surgery* 14(1):9–12.

Dalkowski A, Fimmel S, Beutler C, Zouboulis ChC (2003). Cryotherapy modifies synthetic activity and differentiation of keloidal fibroblasts *in vitro*. *Experimental Dermatology* 12(5):673–681.

Dzubow LM, Miller WH Jr (1987). The effect of 13-cis-retinoic acid on wound healing in dogs. *Journal of Dermatologic Surgery and Oncology* 13(3):265–268.

El-Domyati MB, Attia SK, Saleh FY, Ahmad HM, Uitto JJ (2004). Trichloroacetic acid peeling versus dermabrasion: a histometric, immunohistochemical, and ultrastructural comparison. *Dermatologic Surgery* 30(2 Pt 1):179–188.

Fisher GH, Kim KH, Bernstein LJ, Geronemus RG (2005). Concurrent use of a handheld forced cold air device minimizes patient discomfort during fractional photothermolysis. *Dermatologic Surgery* 31:1242–1243.

Fujiwara M, Muragaki Y, Ooshima A (2005). Upregulation of transforming growth factor-beta1 and vascular endothelial growth factor in cultured keloid fibroblasts: relevance to angiogenic activity. *Archives for Dermatological Research* 297(4):161–169.

Friedman PM, Geronemus RG (2000). Antibiotic prophylaxes in laser resurfacing patients. *Dermatologic Surgery* 26:695–697.

Garden JM, O'Banion MK, Bakus AD, Olson C (2002). Viral disease transmitted by laser-generated plume (aerosol). *Archives of Dermatology* 138:1303–1307.

Gaspar Z, Vinciullo C, Elliott T (2001). Antibiotic prophylaxis for full-face laser resurfacing: is it necessary? *Archives of Dermatology* 137:313–315.

Gold MH, Foster TD, Adair MA, Burlison K, Lewis T (2001). Prevention of hypertrophic scars and keloids by the prophylactic use of topical silicone gel sheets following a surgical procedure in an office setting. *Dermatologic Surgery* 27(7):641–644.

Goldberg DJ, Amin S, Hussain M (2006). Acne scar correction using calcium hydroxylapatite in a carrier-based gel. *Journal of Cosmetic and Laser Therapy* 8(3):134–136.

Gonzalez MJ, Sturgill WH, Ross EV, Uebelhoer NS (2008). Treatment of acne scars using the plasma skin regeneration (PSR) system. *Lasers in Surgery and Medicine* 40(2):124–127.

Hasegawa T, Matsukura T, Mizuno Y, Suga Y, Ogawa H, Ikeda S (2006). Clinical trial of a laser device called fractional photothermolysis system for acne scars. *Journal of Dermatology* 33(9):623–627.

Jacob CI, Dover JS, Kaminer MS (2001). Acne scarring: a classification system and review of treatment options. *Journal of the American Academy of Dermatology* 45(1):109–117.

Jacob SE, Berman B, Nassiri M, Vincek V (2003). Topical application of imiquimod 5% cream to keloids alters expression genes associated with apoptosis. *British Journal of Dermatology* 149(Suppl 66):62–65.

Jeong JT, Kye YC (2001). Resurfacing of pitted facial acne scars with a long-pulsed Er:YAG laser. *Dermatologic Surgery* 27(2):107–110.

Kauh YC, Rouda S, Mondragon G, *et al.* (1997). Major suppression of pro-alpha1(I) type I collagen gene expression in the dermis after keloid excision and immediate intrawound injection of triamcinolone acetonide. *Journal of the American Academy of Dermatology* 37(4):586–589.

Katz BE, Mac Farlane DF (1994). Atypical facial scarring after isotretinoin therapy in a patient with previous dermabrasion. *Journal of the American Academy of Dermatology* 30(5 Pt 2):852–853.

Kilmer S, Semchyshyn N, Shah G, Fitzpatrick R (2007). A pilot study on the use of a plasma skin regeneration device (Portrait PSR3) in full facial rejuvenation procedures. *Lasers in Medical Science* 22(2):101–109.

Klein AW (2006). Soft tissue augmentation 2006: filler fantasy. *Dermatologic Therapy* 19(3):129–133.

Kuo YR, Jeng SF, Wang FS, *et al.* (2004). Flashlamp pulsed-dye laser (PDL) suppression of keloid proliferation through down-regulation of TGF-beta1 expression and extracellular matrix expression. *Lasers in Surgery and Medicine* 34(2):104–108.

Kuo YR, Wu WS, Jeng SF, *et al.* (2005). Suppressed TGF-beta1 expression is correlated with up-regulation of matrix metalloproteinase-13 in keloid regression after flashlamp pulsed-dye laser treatment. *Lasers in Surgery and Medicine* 36(1):38–42.

Kuo YR, Wu WS, Wang FS (2007). Flashlamp pulsed-dye laser suppressed TGF-beta1 expression and proliferation in cultured keloid fibroblasts is mediated by MAPK pathway. *Lasers in Surgery and Medicine* 39(4):358–364.

Laubach HJ, Tannous Z, Anderson RR, Manstein D (2006). Skin responses to fractional photothermolysis. *Lasers in Surgery and Medicine* 38:142–149.

Lee JB, Chung WG, Kwahck H, Lee KH (2002). Focal treatment of acne scars with trichloroacetic acid: chemical reconstruction of skin scars method. *Dermatologic Surgery* 28(11):1017–1021.

Lee KS, Song JY, Suh MH (1991). Collagen mRNA expression detected by *in situ* hybridization in keloid tissue. *Journal of Dermatological Science* 2(4):316–323.

Lupo MP (2006). Hyaluronic acid fillers in facial rejuvenation. *Seminars in Cutaneous Medicine and Surgery* 25(3):122–126.

Manstein D, Herron GS, Sink RK, Tanner H, Anderson RR (2004). Fractional photothermolysis: a new concept for cutaneous remodeling using microscopic patterns of thermal injury. *Lasers in Surgery and Medicine* 34:426–438.

Manuskiatti W, Fitzpatrick RE, Goldman MP, Krejci-Papa N (1999). Prophylactic antibiotics in patients undergoing laser resurfacing of the skin. *Journal of the American Academy of Dermatology* 40:77–84.

Matarasso SL (2006). The use of injectable collagens for aesthetic rejuvenation. *Seminars in Cutaneous Medicine and Surgery* 25(3):151–157.

Majid I (2009) Microneedling therapy in atrophic facial scars: an objective assessment. *Journal of Cutaneous and Aesthetic Surgery* 2(1):26–30.

Monheit GD (1995). Facial resurfacing may trigger the herpes simplex virus. *Cosmetic Dermatology* 8:9–16.

Monheit GD, Coleman KM (2006). Hyaluronic acid fillers. *Dermatologic Therapy* 19(3):141–150.

Nagy IZ, Toth VN, Verzar F (1974). High-resolution electron microscopy of thermal collagen denaturation in tail tendons of young, adult, and old rats. *Connective Tissue Research* 2:265–272.

Nanni CA, Alster TS (1998). Complications of carbon dioxide laser resurfacing. An evaluation of 500 patients. *Dermatologic Surgery* 24:315–320.

Oh J, Kim N, Seo S, Kim IH (2007). Alteration of extracellular matrix modulators after nonablative laser therapy in skin rejuvenation. *British Journal of Dermatology* 157(2):306–310.

Ogawa R, Miyashita T, Hyakusoku H, Akaishi S, Kuribayashi S, Tateno A (2007). Postoperative radiation protocol for keloids and hypertrophic scars: statistical analysis of 370 sites followed for over 18 months. *Annals of Plastic Surgery* 59(6):688–691.

Ogawa R, Yoshitatsu S, Yoshida K, Miyashita T (2009). Is radiation therapy for keloids acceptable? The risk of radiation-induced carcinogenesis. *Plastic and Reconstructive Surgery* 124(4):1196–1201.

Ong CT, Khoo YT, Tan EK, *et al.* (2007). Epithelial–mesenchymal interactions in keloid pathogenesis modulate vascular endothelial growth factor expression and secretion. *Journal of Pathology* 211(1):95–108.

Orentreich DS, Orentreich N (1995). Subcutaneous incisionless (subcision) surgery for the correction of depressed scars and wrinkles. *Dermatologic Surgery* 21(6):543–549.

Orringer JS, Voorhees JJ, Hamilton T (2005). Dermal matrix remodeling after nonablative laser therapy. *Journal of the American Academy of Dermatology* 53(5):775–782.

Rahman Z, Alam M, Dover JS (2006). Fractional laser treatment for pigmentation and texture improvement. *Skin Therapy Letter* 11(9):7–11.

Rogachefsky AS, Hussain M, Goldberg DJ (2003). Atrophic and a mixed pattern of acne scars improved with a 1320 nm Nd:YAG laser. *Dermatologic Surgery* 29(9):904–908.

Rosenberg GJ, Brito MA Jr, Aportella R, Kapoor S (1999). Long-term histologic effects of the CO_2 laser. *Plastic and Reconstructive Surgery* 104:2239–2244.

Ross EV, Amesbury EC, Barile A, Proctor-Shipman L, Feldman BD (1998). Incidence of postoperative infection or positive culture after facial laser resurfacing: a pilot study, a case report, and a proposal for a rational approach to antibiotic prophylaxis. *Journal of the American Academy of Dermatology* 39:975–981.

Ross EV, Swann M, Soon S, Izadpanah A, Barnette D, Davenport S (2009). Full-face treatments with the 2790 nm erbium:YSGG laser system. *Journal of Drugs in Dermatology* 8(3):248–252.

Rubenstein R, Roenigk HH Jr, Stegman SJ, Hanke CW (1986). Atypical keloids after dermabrasion of patients taking isotretinoin. *Journal of the American Academy of Dermatology* 15(2 Pt 1):280–285.

Sharma S, Bhanot A, Kaur A, Dewan SP (2007). Role of liquid nitrogen alone compared with combination of liquid nitrogen and intralesional triamcinolone acetonide in treatment of small keloids. *Journal of Cosmetic Dermatology* **6**(4):258–261.

Stegman SJ (1982). A comparative histologic study of the effects of three peeling agents and dermabrasion on normal and sundamaged skin. *Aesthetic Plastic Surgery* **6**(3):123–135.

Tanzi EL, Alster TS (2003a). Single-pass carbon dioxide versus multiple-pass Er:YAG laser skin resurfacing: a comparison of postoperative wound healing and side-effect rates. *Dermatologic Surgery* **29**(1):80–84.

Tanzi EL, Alster TS (2003b). Side effects and complications of variable-pulsed erbium:yttrium-aluminum-garnet laser skin resurfacing: extended experience with 50 patients. *Plastic and Reconstructive Surgery* **111**: 1524–1529.

Tanzi EL, Alster TS (2004). Comparison of a 1450 nm diode laser and a 1320 nm Nd:YAG laser in the treatment of atrophic facial scars: a prospective clinical and histologic study. *Dermatologic Surgery* **30**(2 Pt 1):152–157.

Teikemeier G, Goldberg DJ (1997). Skin resurfacing with the erbium:YAG laser. *Dermatologic Surgery* **23**:685–687.

Tsukahara K, Takema Y, Moriwaki S, Fujimura T, Imayama S, Imokawa G (2001). Carbon dioxide laser treatment promotes repair of the three-dimensional network of elastic fibres in rat skin. *British Journal of Dermatology* **144**:452–458.

Tzikas TL (2008). A 52 month summary of results using calcium hydroxylapatite for facial soft tissue augmentation. *Dermatologic Surgery* **34**(1 Suppl):S9–S15.

Uitto J, Perejda AJ, Abergel RP, Chu ML, Ramirez F (1985). Altered steady-state ratio of type I/III procollagen mRNAs correlates with selectively increased type I procollagen biosynthesis in cultured keloid fibroblasts. *Proceedings of the National Academy of Sciences USA* **82**(17):5935–5939.

Varnavides CK, Forster RA, Cunliffe WJ (1987). The role of bovine collagen in the treatment of acne scars. *British Journal of Dermatology* **116**(2):199–206.

Verzar F, Nagy IZ (1970). Electronmicroscopic analysis of thermal collagen denaturation in rat tail tendons. *Gerontologia* **16**:77–82.

Walia S, Alster TS (1999a). Prolonged clinical and histologic effects from CO_2 laser resurfacing of atrophic acne scars. *Dermatologic Surgery* **25**(12):926–930.

Walia S, Alster TS (1999b). Cutaneous CO_2 laser resurfacing infection rate with and without prophylactic antibiotics. *Dermatologic Surgery* **25**(12):857–861.

Weinstein C (1999). Erbium laser resurfacing: current concepts. *Plastic and Reconstructive Surgery* **103**:602–616.

West TB, Alster TS (1999). Effect of pretreatment on the incidence of hyperpigmentation following cutaneous CO_2 laser resurfacing. *Dermatologic Surgery* **25**:15–17.

Wolfram D, Tzankov A, Pulzl P, Piza-Katzer H (2009). Hypertrophic scars and keloids – a review of their pathophysiology, risk factors, and therapeutic management. *Dermatologic Surgery* **35**(2):171–181.

Yosipovitch G, Widijanti Sugeng M, Goon A, Chan YH, Goh CL (2001). A comparison of the combined effect of cryotherapy and corticosteroid injections versus corticosteroids and cryotherapy alone on keloids: a controlled study. *Journal of Dermatological Treatment* **12**(2):87–90.

Younai S, Venters G, Vu S, Nichter L, Nimni ME, Tuan TL (1996). Role of growth factors in scar contraction: an *in vitro* analysis. *Annals of Plastic Surgery* **36**(5):495–501.

Yug A, Lane JE, Howard MS, Kent DE (2006). Histologic study of depressed acne scars treated with serial high-concentration (95%) trichloroacetic acid. *Dermatologic Surgery* **32**(8):985–990.

Zachariae H (1988). Delayed wound healing and keloid formation following argon laser treatment or dermabrasion during isotretinoin treatment. *British Journal of Dermatology* **118**(5):703–706.

Zachary CB (2000). Modulating the Er:YAG laser. *Lasers in Surgery and Medicine* **26**:223–226.

Chapter 5

Akamatsu H, Oguchi M, Nishijima S, *et al.* (1990). The inhibition of free radical generation by human neutrophils through the synergistic effects of metronidazole with palmitoleic acid: a possible mechanism of action of metronidazole in rosacea and acne. *Archives of Dermatological Research* **282**(7):449–454.

Akpek EK, Merchant A, Pinar V, Foster CS (1997). Ocular rosacea: patient characteristics and follow-up. *Ophthalmology* **104**(11):1863–1867.

Aloi F, Tomasini C, Soro E, Pippione M (2000). The clinicopathologic spectrum of rhinophyma. *Journal of the American Academy of Dermatology* **42**(3):468–472.

Andrews JR (1982). The prevalence of hair follicle mites in caucasian New Zealanders. *New Zealand Medical Journal* **95**(711):451–453.

Bamford JT, Tilden RL, Blankush JL, Gangeness DE (1999). Effect of treatment of *Helicobacter pylori* infection on rosacea. *Archives of Dermatology* **135**(6):659–663.

Bamford JT, Gessert CE, Renier CM, *et al.* (2006). Childhood stye and adult rosacea. *Journal of the American Academy of Dermatology* **55**(6):951–955.

Berg M, Liden S (1989). An epidemiological study of rosacea. *Acta Dermato-Venereologica* **69**(5):419–423.

Bevins CL, Liu FT (2007). Rosacea: skin innate immunity gone awry? *Nature Medicine* **13**(8):904–906.

Bonnar E, Eustace P, Powell FC (1993). The *Demodex* mite population in rosacea. *Journal of the American Academy of Dermatology* **28**(3):443–448.

Borrie P (1955a). The state of the blood vessels of the face in rosacea. I. *British Journal of Dermatology* **67**(1):5–8.

Borrie P (1955b). The state of the blood vessels of the face in rosacea. II. *British Journal of Dermatology* **67**(2):73–75.

Brinnel H, Friedel J, Caputa M, Cabanac M, Grosshans E (1989). Rosacea: disturbed defense against brain overheating. *Archives of Dermatological Research* **281**(1):66–72.

Browning DJ, Proia AD (1986). Ocular rosacea. *Survey of Ophthalmology* **31**:145–158.

Chamaillard M, Mortemousque B, Boralevi F (2008). Cutaneous and ocular signs of childhood rosacea. *Archives of Dermatology* **144**(2):167–171.

Chen DM, Crosby DL (1997). Periorbital edema as an initial presentation of rosacea. *Journal of the American Academy of Dermatology* **37**:346–348.

Crawford GH, Pelle MT, James WD (2004). Rosacea: I. Etiology, pathogenesis, and subtype classification. *Journal of the American Academy of Dermatology* **51**:327–341.

Crosti C, Menni S, Sala F, Piccinno R (1983). Demodectic infestation of the pilosebaceous follicle. *Journal of Cutaneous Pathology* **10**(4):257–261.

Curnier A, Choudhary S (2004). Rhinophyma: dispelling the myths. *Plastic and Reconstructive Surgery* **114**(2):351–354.

Dahl MV (2001). Pathogenesis of rosacea. *Advances in Dermatology* **17**:29–45.

Dan L, Shi-long Y, Miao-li L, *et al.* (2008). Inhibitory effect of oral doxycycline on neovascularization in a rat corneal alkali burn model of angiogenesis. *Current Eye Research* **33**(8):653–660.

Di Nardo A, Yamasaki K, Dorschner RA, Lai Y, Gallo RL (2008). Mast cell cathelicidin antimicrobial peptide prevents invasive group A *Streptococcus* infection of the skin. *Journal of Immunology* **180**(11):7565–7573.

Drolet B, Paller AS (1992). Childhood rosacea. *Pediatric Dermatology* 9(1):22–26.

Ecker RI, Winkelmann RK (1979). *Demodex* granuloma. *Archives of Dermatology* 115(3):343–344.

Engel A, Johnson ML, Haynes SG (1988). Health effects of sunlight exposure in the United States. Results from the first National Health and Nutrition Examination Survey, 1971–1974. *Archives of Dermatology* 124(1):72–79.

[2Erbagci Z, Ozgoztasi O (1998). The significance of *Demodex folliculorum* density in rosacea. *International Journal of Dermatology* 37(6):421–425.

Erzurum SA, Feder RS, Greenwald MJ (1993). Acne rosacea with keratitis in childhood. *Archives of Ophthalmology* 111(2):228–230.

Fife RS, Sledge GW Jr, Sissons S, Zerler B (2000). Effects of tetracyclines on angiogenesis *in vitro*. *Cancer Letters* 153(1–2):75–78.

Fisher GJ, Talwar HS, Lin J, Voorhees JJ (1999). Molecular mechanisms of photoaging in human skin *in vivo* and their prevention by all-trans retinoic acid. *Photochemistry and Photobiology* 69(2):154–157.

Forton F (1986). *Demodex* et inflammation perifolliculaire chez l'homme: revue et observation de 69 biopsies. *Annales de Dermatologie et de Vénéréologie* 113(11):1047–1058.

Forton F, Seys B (1993). Density of *Demodex folliculorum* in rosacea: a case-control study using standardized skin-surface biopsy. *British Journal of Dermatology* 128(6):650–659.

Freeman BS (1970). Reconstructive rhinoplasty for rhinophyma. *Plastic and Reconstructive Surgery* 46(3):265–270.

Gedik GK, Karaduman A, Sivri B, Caner B (2005). Has *Helicobacter pylori* eradication therapy any effect on severity of rosacea symptoms? *Journal of the European Academy of Dermatology and Venereology* 19(3):398–399.

Gilbertson-Beadling S, Powers EA, Stamp-Cole M, *et al.* (1995). The tetracycline analogs minocycline and doxycycline inhibit angiogenesis *in vitro* by a non-metalloproteinase-dependent mechanism. *Cancer Chemotherapy and Pharmacology* 36(5):418–424.

Gomaa AH, Yaar M, Eyada MM, Bhawan J (2007). Lymphangiogenesis and angiogenesis in non-phymatous rosacea. *Journal of Cutaneous Pathology* 34(10):748–753.

Greaves MW, Burova E (1997). Flushing: causes, investigation and clinical consequences. *Journal of the European Academy of Dermatology and Venereology* 8(2):91–100.

Guzman-Sanchez DA, Ishiuji Y, Patel T, Fountain J, Chan YH, Yosipovitch G (2007). Enhanced skin blood flow and sensitivity to noxious heat stimuli in papulopustular rosacea. *Journal of the American Academy of Dermatology* 57(5):800–805.

Harvey DT, Fenske NA, Glass LF (1998). Rosaceous lymphedema: a rare variant of a common disorder. *Cutis* 61:321–324.

Helm KF, Menz J, Gibson LE, Dicken CH (1991). A clinical and histopathologic study of granulomatous rosacea. *Journal of the American Academy of Dermatology* 25 (6 Pt 1):1038–1043.

Herr H, You CH (2000). Relationship between *Helicobacter pylori* and rosacea: it may be a myth. *Journal of Korean Medical Science* 15(5):551–554.

Higgins E, du Vivier A (1999). Alcohol intake and other skin disorders. *Clinical Dermatology* 17(4):437–441.

Hoekzema R, Hulsebosch HJ, Bos JD (1995). Demodicidosis or rosacea: what did we treat? *British Journal of Dermatology* 133(2):294–299.

Howell MD, Jones JF, Kisich KO, Streib JE, Gallo RL, Leung DY (2004). Selective killing of vaccinia virus by LL-37: implications for eczema vaccinatum. *Journal of Immunology* 172(3):1763–1767.

Jansen T, Plewig G (1998). Clinical and histological variants of rhinophyma, including nonsurgical treatment modalities. *Facial Plastic Surgery* 14:241–253.

Jappe U, Schnuch A, Uter W (2005). Rosacea and contact allergy to cosmetics and topical medicaments–retrospective analysis of multicentre surveillance data 1995–2002. *Contact Dermatitis* 52(2):96–101.

Jones D (2004). Reactive oxygen species and rosacea. *Cutis* 74(3 Suppl):17–20, 32–34.

Jones MP, Knable AL Jr, White MJ, Durning SJ (1998). *Helicobacter pylori* in rosacea: lack of an association. *Archives of Dermatology* 134(4):511.

Kligman AM (2006). An experimental critique on the state of knowledge of rosacea. *Journal of Cosmetic Dermatology* 5:76–80.

Koczulla R, von Degenfeld G, Kupatt C, *et al.* (2003). An angiogenic role for the human peptide antibiotic LL-37/hCAP-18. *Journal of Clinical Investigation* 111(11):1665–1672.

Kyriakis KP, Palamaras I, Terzoudi S, Emmanuelides S, Michailides C, Pagana G (2005). Epidemiologic aspects of rosacea. *Journal of the American Academy of Dermatology* 53(5):918–919.

Lacey N, Delaney S, Kavanagh K, Powell FC (2007). Mite-related bacterial antigens stimulate inflammatory cells in rosacea. *British Journal of Dermatology* 157(3):474–481.

Lee M, Koo J (2005). Rosacea, light, and phototherapy. *Journal of Drugs in Dermatology* 4(3):326–329.

Lemp MA, Mahmood MA, Weiler HH (1984). Association of rosacea and keratoconjunctivitis sicca. *Archives of Ophthalmology* 102(4):556–557.

Lonne-Rahm SB, Fischer T, Berg M (1999). Stinging and rosacea. *Acta Dermato-Venereologica* 79(6):460–461.

Marks R, Harcourt-Webster JN (1969). Histopathology of rosacea. *Archives of Dermatology* 100(6):683–691.

Marks R, Jones EW (1969). Disseminated rosacea. *British Journal of Dermatology* 81(1):16–28.

Millikan LE (2004). Rosacea as an inflammatory disorder: a unifying theory? *Cutis* 73(1 Suppl):5–8.

Neumann E, Frithz A (1998). Capillaropathy and capillaroneogenesis in the pathogenesis of rosacea. *Internation Journal of Dermatology* 37(4):263–266.

Nizet V, Ohtake T, Lauth X, *et al.* (2001). Innate antimicrobial peptide protects the skin from invasive bacterial infection. *Nature* 414(6862):454–457.

Oztas MO, Balk M, Ogus E, Bozkurt M, Ogus IH, Ozer N (2003). The role of free oxygen radicals in the aetiopathogenesis of rosacea. *Clinical and Experimental Dermatology* 28(2):188–192.

Ramelet AA, Perroulaz G (1988). Rosacea: histopathologic study of 75 cases. *Annales de Dermatologie et de Vénéréologie* 115(8):801–806.

Rebora A, Drago F, Parodi A (1995). May *Helicobacter pylori* be important for dermatologists? *Dermatology* 191(1):6–8.

Rohrich RJ, Griffin JR, Adams WP Jr (2002). Rhinophyma: review and update. *Plastic and Reconstructive Surgery* 110(3):860–869.

Rosenberger CM, Gallo RL, Finlay BB (2004). Interplay between antibacterial effectors: a macrophage antimicrobial peptide impairs intracellular *Salmonella* replication. *Proceedings of the National Academy of Sciences of the United States of America* 101(8):2422–2427.

Scerri L, Saihan EM (1995). Persistent facial swelling in a patient with rosacea. Rosacea lymphedema. *Archives of Dermatology* 131(9):1071, 1074.

Sharma VK, Lynn A, Kaminski M, Vasudeva R, Howden CW (1998). A study of the prevalence of *Helicobacter pylori* infection and other markers of upper gastrointestinal tract disease in patients with rosacea. *American Journal of Gastroenterology* 93(2):220–222.

Starr PA, Macdonald A (1969). Oculocutaneous aspects of rosacea. *Proceedings of the Royal Society of Medicine* 62(1):9–11.

Szlachcic A, Sliwowski Z, Karczewska E, Bielanski W, Pytko-Polonczyk J, Konturek SJ (1999). *Helicobacter pylori* and its eradication in rosacea. *Journal of Physiology and Pharmacology* 50(5):777–786.

Tur E, Tur M, Maibach HI, Guy RH (1983). Basal perfusion of the cutaneous microcirculation: measurements as a function of anatomic position. *Journal of Investigative Dermatology* 81(5):442–446.

Utas S, Ozbakir O, Turasan A, Utas C (1999). *Helicobacter pylori* eradication treatment reduces the severity of rosacea. *Journal of the American Academy of Dermatology* 40(3):433–435.

van de Scheur MR, van der Waal RI, Starink TM (2003). Lupus miliaris disseminatus faciei: a distinctive rosacea-like syndrome and not a granulomatous form of rosacea. *Dermatology* 206(2):120–123.

Wilkin JK (1981). Oral thermal-induced flushing in erythematotelangiectatic rosacea. *Journal of Investigative Dermatology* 76:15–18.

Wilkin JK (1988). Why is flushing limited to a mostly facial cutaneous distribution? *Journal of the American Academy of Dermatology* 19(2 Pt 1):309–313.

Wilkin JK (1994). Rosacea. Pathophysiology and treatment. *Archives of Dermatology* 130(3):359–362.

Wilkin J, Dahl M, Detmar M, *et al.* (2002). Standard classification of rosacea: report of the National Rosacea Society Expert Committee on the classification and staging of rosacea. *Journal of the American Academy of Dermatology* 46(4):584–587.

Yamasaki K, Schauber J, Coda A, *et al.* (2006). Kallikrein-mediated proteolysis regulates the antimicrobial effects of cathelicidins in skin. *FASEB Journal* 20(12):2068–2080.

Yamasaki K, Di Nardo A, Bardan A, *et al.* (2007). Increased serine protease activity and cathelicidin promotes skin inflammation in rosacea. *Nature Medicine* 13(8):975–980.

Yang D, Chen Q, Schmidt AP, *et al.* (2000). LL-37, the neutrophil granule- and epithelial cell-derived cathelicidin, utilizes formyl peptide receptor-like 1 (FPRL1) as a receptor to chemoattract human peripheral blood neutrophils, monocytes, and T cells. *Journal of Experimental Medicine* 192(7):1069–1074.

Yano K, Kadoya K, Kajiya K, Hong YK, Detmar M (2005). Ultraviolet B irradiation of human skin induces an angiogenic switch that is mediated by upregulation of vascular endothelial growth factor and by downregulation of thrombospondin-1. *British Journal of Dermatology* 152(1):115–121.

Yazici AC, Tamer L, Ikizoglu G, *et al.* (2006). GSTM1 and GSTT1 null genotypes as possible heritable factors of rosacea. *Photodermatology, Photoimmunology and Photomedicine* 22(4):208–210.

Chapter 6

Aizawa H, Niimura M, Kon Y (1992). Influence of oral metronidazole on the endocrine milieu and sebum excretion rate. *Journal of Dermatology* 19(12):959–963.

Akamatsu H, Oguchi M, Nishijima S, *et al.* (1990). The inhibition of free radical generation by human neutrophils through the synergistic effects of metronidazole with palmitoleic acid: a possible mechanism of action of metronidazole in rosacea and acne. *Archives of Dermatological Research* 282(7):449–454.

Akamatsu H, Komura J, Asada Y, Miyachi Y, Niwa Y (1991). Inhibitory effect of azelaic acid on neutrophil functions: a possible cause for its efficacy in treating pathogenetically unrelated diseases. *Archives of Dermatological Research* 283(3):162–166.

Akamatsu H, Asada M, Komura J, Asada Y, Niwa Y (1992). Effect of doxycycline on the generation of reactive oxygen species: a possible mechanism of action of acne therapy with doxycycline. *Acta Dermato-Venereologica* 72(3):178–179.

Altinyazar HC, Koca R, Tekin NS, Esturk E (2005). Adapalene *vs.* metronidazole gel for the treatment of rosacea. *International Journal of Dermatology* 44(3):252–255.

Amin AR, Attur MG, Thakker GD, *et al.* (1996). A novel mechanism of action of tetracyclines: effects on nitric oxide synthases. *Proceedings of the National Academy of Sciences of the United States of America* 93(24):14014–14019.

Bakar O, Demircay Z, Yuksel M, Haklar G, Sanisoglu Y (2007). The effect of azithromycin on reactive oxygen species in rosacea. *Clinical and Experimental Dermatology* 32(2):197–200.

Bendesky A, Menendez D, Ostrosky-Wegman P (2002). Is metronidazole carcinogenic? *Mutation Research* 511(2):133–144.

Berger R, Barba A, Fleischer A, *et al.* (2007). A double-blinded, randomized, vehicle-controlled, multicenter, parallel-group study to assess the safety and efficacy of tretinoin gel microsphere 0.04% in the treatment of acne vulgaris in adults. *Cutis* 80(2):152–157.

Bjerke R, Fyrand O, Graupe K (1999). Double-blind comparison of azelaic acid 20% cream and its vehicle in treatment of papulo-pustular rosacea. *Acta Dermato-Venereologica* 79(6):456–459.

Camisa C, Eisenstat B, Ragaz A, Weissmann G (1982). The effects of retinoids on neutrophil functions *in vitro*. *Journal of the American Academy of Dermatology* 6(4 Pt 2 Suppl):620–629.

Cho DH, Choi YJ, Jo SA, Nam JH, Jung SC, Jo I (2005). Retinoic acid decreases nitric oxide production in endothelial cells: a role of phosphorylation of endothelial nitric oxide synthase at Ser(1179). *Biochemical and Biophysical Research Communications* 326(4):703–710.

Choudry K, Beck MH, Muston HL (2002). Allergic contact dermatitis from 2-bromo-2-nitropropane-1, 3-diol in Metrogel. *Contact Dermatitis* 46(1):60–61.

Dahl MV, Katz HI, Krueger GG, *et al.* (1998). Topical metronidazole maintains remissions of rosacea. *Archives of Dermatology* 134(6):679–683.

Dahl MV (2001). Pathogenesis of rosacea. *Advances in Dermatology* 17:29–45.

Del Rosso JQ (2005). Adjunctive skin care in the management of rosacea: cleansers, moisturizers, and photoprotectants. *Cutis* 75(3 Suppl):17–21.

Draelos ZD (2004). Facial hygiene and comprehensive management of rosacea. *Cutis* 73(3):183–187.

Draelos ZD (2006a). The effect of Cetaphil Gentle Skin Cleanser on the skin barrier of patients with rosacea. *Cutis* 77(4 Suppl):27–33.

Draelos ZD (2006b). The rationale for advancing the formulation of azelaic acid vehicles. *Cutis* 77(2 Suppl):7–11.

Draelos ZD (2008). Optimizing redness reduction, part 2: rosacea and cosmeceuticals. *Cosmetic Dermatology* 21(8):433–436.

Elewski BE, Fleischer AB Jr, Pariser DM (2003). A comparison of 15% azelaic acid gel and 0.75% metronidazole gel in the topical treatment of papulopustular rosacea: results of a randomized trial. *Archives of Dermatology* 139(11):1444–1450.

Elewski BE (2007). Percutaneous absorption kinetics of topical metronidazole formulations *in vitro* in the human cadaver skin model. *Advances in Therapy* 24(2):239–246.

Engel A, Johnson ML, Haynes SG (1988). Health effects of sunlight exposure in the United States. Results from the first National Health and Nutrition Examination Survey, 1971–1974. *Archives of Dermatology* 124(1):72–79.

Erdogan FG, Yurtsever P, Aksoy D, Eskioglu F (1998). Efficacy of low-dose isotretinoin in patients with treatment-resistant rosacea. *Archives of Dermatology* 134(7):884–885.

Ertl GA, Levine N, Kligman AM (1994). A comparison of the efficacy of topical tretinoin and low-dose oral isotretinoin in rosacea. *Archives of Dermatology* 130(3):319–324.

Esterly NB, Furey NL, Flanagan LE (1978). The effect of antimicrobial agents on leukocyte chemotaxis. *Journal of Investigative Dermatology* 70(1):51–55.

Esterly NB, Koransky JS, Furey NL, Trevisan M (1984). Neutrophil chemotaxis in patients with acne receiving oral tetracycline therapy. *Archives of Dermatology* 120(10):1308–1313.

Falcon RH, Lee WL, Shalita AR, Suntharalingam K, Fikrig SM (1986). *In vitro* effect of isotretinoin on monocyte chemotaxis. *Journal of Investigative Dermatology* 86(5):550–552.

[Fernandez-Obregon A (1994). Oral use of azithromycin for the treatment of acne rosacea. *Archives of Dermatology* 140(4):489–490.

Golub LM, Sorsa T, Lee HM (1995). Doxycycline inhibits neutrophil (PMN)-type matrix metalloproteinases in human adult periodontitis gingiva. *Journal of Clinical Periodontology* 22(2):100–109.

Guerin C, Laterra J, Masnyk T, Golub LM, Brem H (1992). Selective endothelial growth inhibition by tetracyclines that inhibit collagenase. *Biochemical and Biophysical Research Communications* 188(2):740–745.

Hofer T (2004). Continuous 'microdose' isotretinoin in adult recalcitrant rosacea. *Clinical and Experimental Dermatology* 29(2):204–205.

Hoting E, Paul E, Plewig G (1986). Treatment of rosacea with isotretinoin. *International Journal of Dermatology* 25(10):660–663.

Ianaro A, Ialenti A, Maffia P, et al. (2000). Anti-inflammatory activity of macrolide antibiotics. *Journal of Pharmacology and Experimental Therapeutics* 292(1):156–163.

Jansen T, Plewig G, Kligman AM (1994). Diagnosis and treatment of rosacea fulminans. *Dermatology* 188(4):251–254.

Jansen T, Plewig G (1998). Clinical and histological variants of rhinophyma, including nonsurgical treatment modalities. *Facial Plastic Surgery* 14(4):241–253.

Kadota J, Iwashita T, Matsubara Y, et al. (1998). Inhibitory effect of erythromycin on superoxide anion production by human neutrophils primed with granulocyte-colony stimulating factor. *Antimicrobial Agents and Chemotherapy* 42(7):1866–1867.

Kligman AM (2006). An experimental critique on the state of knowledge of rosacea. *Journal of Cosmetic Dermatology* 5:76–80.

Kloppenburg M, Verweij CL, Miltenburg AM, et al. (1995). The influence of tetracyclines on T cell activation. *Clinical and Experimental Immunology* 102(3):635–641.

Labro MT (1998). Anti-inflammatory activity of macrolides: a new therapeutic potential? *Journal of Antimicrobial Chemotherapy* 41(Suppl B):37–46.

Lachgar S, Charveron M, Gall Y, Bonafe JL (1999). Inhibitory effects of retinoids on vascular endothelial growth factor production by cultured human skin keratinocytes. *Dermatology* 199(1 Suppl):25–27.

Lamp KC, Freeman CD, Klutman NE, Lacy MK (1999). Pharmacokinetics and pharmacodynamics of the nitroimidazole antimicrobials. *Clinical Pharmacokinetics* 36(5):353–373.

Laquieze S, Czernielewski J, Baltas E (2007). Beneficial use of Cetaphil moisturizing cream as part of a daily skin care regimen for individuals with rosacea. *Journal of Dermatological Treatment* 18(3):158–162.

Lebwohl MG, Medansky RS, Russo CL, Plott RT (1995). The comparative efficacy of sodium sulfacetamide 10%/sulfur 5% (Sulfacet-R) lotion and metronidazole 0.75% (MetroGel) in the treatment of rosacea. *Journal of Geriatric Dermatology* 3(5):183–185.

Lee JY, Mak CP, Wang BJ, Chang WC (1992). Effects of retinoids on endothelial cell proliferation, prostacyclin production and platelet aggregation. *Journal of Dermatological Science* 3(3):157–162.

Lee M, Koo J (2005). Rosacea, light, and phototherapy. *Journal of Drugs in Dermatology* 4(3):326–329.

Levert H, Gressier B, Moutard I, et al. (1998). Azithromycin impact on neutrophil oxidative metabolism depends on exposure time. *Inflammation* 22(2):191–201.

Liu PT, Krutzik SR, Kim J, Modlin RL (2005). Cutting edge: all-trans retinoic acid down-regulates TLR2 expression and function. *Journal of Immunology* 174(5):2467–2470.

Lonne-Rahm SB, Fischer T, Berg M (1999). Stinging and rosacea. *Acta Dermato-Venereologica* 79(6):460–461.

Maddin S (1999). A comparison of topical azelaic acid 20% cream and topical metronidazole 0.75% cream in the treatment of patients with papulopustular rosacea. *Journal of the American Academy of Dermatology* 40(6 Pt 1):961–965.

Madsen JT, Thormann J, Kerre S, Andersen KE, Goossens A (2007). Allergic contact dermatitis to topical metronidazole–3 cases. *Contact Dermatitis* 56(6):364–366.

Martinez V, Caumes E (2001). Metronidazole. *Annales de Dermatologie et de Vénéréologie* 128(8–9):903–909.

Maru U, Michaud P, Garrigue J, Oustrin J, Rouffiac R (1982). *In vitro* diffusion and skin penetration of azelaic preparations: study of correlations. *Journal de Pharmacie de Belgique* 37(3):207–213.

Menendez D, Bendesky A, Rojas E, Salamanca F, Ostrosky-Wegman P (2002). Role of P53 functionality in the genotoxicity of metronidazole and its hydroxy metabolite. *Mutation Research* 501(1–2):57–67.

Miyachi Y, Imamura S, Niwa Y (1986). Anti-oxidant action of metronidazole: a possible mechanism of action in rosacea. *British Journal of Dermatology* 114(2):231–234.

Narayanan S, Hunerbein A, Getie M, Jackel A, Neubert RH (2007). Scavenging properties of metronidazole on free oxygen radicals in a skin lipid model system. *Journal of Pharmacy and Pharmacology* 59(8):1125–1130.

Modi S, Harting M, Rosen T (2008). Azithromycin as an alternative rosacea therapy when tetracyclines prove problematic. *Journal of Drugs in Dermatology* 7(9):898–899.

Nielsen PG (1983). The relapse rate for rosacea after treatment with either oral tetracycline or metronidazole cream. *British Journal of Dermatology* 109(1):122.

Norris DA, Osborn R, Robinson W, Tonnesen MG (1987). Isotretinoin produces significant inhibition of monocyte and neutrophil chemotaxis *in vivo* in patients with cystic acne. *Journal of Investigative Dermatology* 89(1):38–43.

Orfanos CE, Bauer R (1983). Evidence for anti-inflammatory activities of oral synthetic retinoids: experimental findings and clinical experience. *British Journal of Dermatology* 109(25 Suppl):55–60.

Passi S, Picardo M, De Luca C, Breathnach AS, Nazzaro-Porro M (1991a). Scavenging activity of azelaic acid on hydroxyl radicals 'in vitro'. *Free Radical Research Communications* 11(6):329–338.

Passi S, Picardo M, Zompetta C, De Luca C, Breathnach AS, Nazzaro-Porro M (1991b). The oxyradical-scavenging activity of azelaic acid in biological systems. *Free Radical Research Communications* 15(1):17–28.

Pye RJ, Burton JL (1976). Treatment of rosacea by metronidazole. *Lancet* 1(7971):1211–1212.

Sainte-Marie I, Tenaud I, Jumbou O, Dreno B (1999). Minocycline modulation of alpha-MSH production by keratinocytes *in vitro*. *Acta Dermato-Venereologica* 79(4):265–267.

Sapadin AN, Fleischmajer R (2006). Tetracyclines: nonantibiotic properties and their clinical implications. *Journal of the American Academy of Dermatology* 54:258–265.

Sato E, Kato M, Kohno M, Niwano Y (2007). Clindamycin phosphate scavenges hydroxyl radical. *International Journal of Dermatology* 46(11):1185–1187.

Schell H, Vogt HJ, Mack-Hennes A (1987). Treatment of rosacea with isotretinoin. Results of a multicenter trial follow-up. *Zeitschrift fur Hautkrankheiten* 62(15):1123–1124, 1129–1133.

Sehgal VN, Sharma S, Sardana K (2008). Rosacea/acne rosacea: efficacy of combination therapy of azithromycin and topical 0.1% tacrolimus ointment. *Journal of the European Academy of Dermatology and Venereology* 22(11):1366–1368.

Shroot B (1998). Pharmacodynamics and pharmacokinetics of topical adapalene. *Journal of the American Academy of Dermatology* 39(2 Pt 3):S17–S24.

Skov MJ, Quigley JW, Bucks DA (1997). Topical delivery system for tretinoin: research and clinical implications. *Journal of Pharmaceutical Sciences* 86(10):1138–1143.

Tamargo RJ, Bok RA, Brem H (1991). Angiogenesis inhibition by minocycline. *Cancer Research* 51(2):672–675.

Tenaud I, Khammari A, Dreno B (2007). *In vitro* modulation of TLR-2, CD1d, and IL-10 by adapalene on normal human skin and acne inflammatory lesions. *Experimental Dermatology* 16(6):500–506.

Thiboutot D, Thieroff-Ekerdt R, Graupe K (2003). Efficacy and safety of azelaic acid (15%) gel as a new treatment for papulopustular rosacea: results from two vehicle-controlled, randomized phase III studies. *Journal of the American Academy of Dermatology* 48(6):836–845.

Thiboutot DM, Fleischer AB Jr, Del Rosso JQ, Graupe K (2008). Azelaic acid 15% gel once daily versus twice daily in papulopustular rosacea. *Journal of Drugs in Dermatology* **7**(6):541–546.

Torok HM, Webster G, Dunlap FE, Egan N, Jarratt M, Stewart D (2005). Combination sodium sulfacetamide 10% and sulfur 5% cream with sunscreens versus metronidazole 0.75% cream for rosacea. *Cutis* **75**(6):357–363.

Turjanmaa K, Reunala T (1987). Isotretinoin treatment of rosacea. *Acta Dermato-Venereologica* **67**(1):89–91.

Visapaa JP, Tillonen JS, Kaihovaara PS, Salaspuro MP (2002). Lack of disulfiram-like reaction with metronidazole and ethanol. *Annals of Pharmacotherapy* **36**(6):971–974.

Wilkin JK, DeWitt S (1993). Treatment of rosacea: topical clindamycin versus oral tetracycline. *International Journal of Dermatology* **32**(1):65–67.

Wilkin JK (1994). Rosacea. Pathophysiology and treatment. *Archives of Dermatology* **130**(3):359–362.

Williams CS, Woodcock KR (2000). Do ethanol and metronidazole interact to produce a disulfiram-like reaction? *Annals of Pharmacotherapy* **34**(2):255–257.

Yao JS, Chen Y, Zhai W, Xu K, Young WL, Yang GY (2004). Minocycline exerts multiple inhibitory effects on vascular endothelial growth factor-induced smooth muscle cell migration: the role of ERK1/2, PI3K, and matrix metalloproteinases. *Circulation Research* **95**(4):364–371.

Yao JS, Shen F, Young WL, Yang GY (2007). Comparison of doxycycline and minocycline in the inhibition of VEGF-induced smooth muscle cell migration. *Neurochemistry International* **50**(3):524–530.

Yoo J, Reid D C, Kimball AB (2006). Metronidazole in the treatment of rosacea: do formulation, dosing, and concentration matter? *Journal of Drugs in Dermatology* **5**(4):317–319.

Yoshioka A, Miyachi Y, Imamura S, Niwa Y (1986). Anti-oxidant effects of retinoids on inflammatory skin diseases. *Archives of Dermatological Research* **278**(3):177–183.

Ziel K, Yelverton CB, Balkrishnan R, Feldman SR (2005). Cumulative irritation potential of metronidazole gel compared to azelaic acid gel after repeated applications to healthy skin. *Journal of Drugs in Dermatology* **4**(6):727–731.

Chapter 7

Altshuler GB, Anderson RR, Manstein D, Zenzie HH, Smirnov MZ (2001). Extended theory of selective photothermolysis. *Lasers in Surgery and Medicine* **29**(5):416–432.

Angermeier MC (1999). Treatment of facial vascular lesions with intense pulsed light. *Journal of Cutaneous Laser Therapy* **1**(2):95–100.

Anderson RR, Parrish JA (1983). Selective photothermolysis: precise microsurgery by selective absorption of pulsed radiation. *Science* **220**(4596):524–527.

Bernstein EF, Kligman A (2008). Rosacea treatment using the new-generation, high-energy, 595 nm, long pulse-duration pulsed-dye laser. *Lasers in Surgery and Medicine* **40**(4):233–239.

Bryld LE, Jemec GB (2007). Photodynamic therapy in a series of rosacea patients. *Journal of the European Academy of Dermatology and Venereology* **21**(9):1199–1202.

Cassuto DA, Ancona DM, Emanuelli G (2000). Treatment of facial telangiectasias with a diode-pumped Nd:YAG laser at 532 nm. *Journal of Cutaneous Laser Therapy* **2**(3):141–146.

Clark C, Cameron H, Moseley H, Ferguson J, Ibbotson SH (2004). Treatment of superficial cutaneous vascular lesions: experience with the KTP 532 nm laser. *Lasers in Medical Science* **19**(1):1–5.

Clark SM, Lanigan SW, Marks R (2002). Laser treatment of erythema and telangiectasia associated with rosacea. *Lasers in Medical Science* **17**(1):26–33.

Eremia S, Li CY (2002). Treatment of face veins with a cryogen spray variable pulse width 1064 nm Nd:YAG laser: a prospective study of 17 patients. *Dermatologic Surgery* **28**(3):244–247.

Goodman GJ, Roberts S, Bezborodoff A (2002). Studies in long-pulsed potassium titanyl phosphate laser for the treatment of spider naevi and perialar telangiectasia. *Australasian Journal of Dermatology* **43**(1):9–14.

Iyer S, Fitzpatrick RE (2005). Long-pulsed dye laser treatment for facial telangiectasias and erythema: evaluation of a single purpuric pass versus multiple subpurpuric passes. *Dermatologic Surgery* **31**(8 Pt 1):898–903.

Jasim ZF, Woo WK, Handley JM (2004). Long-pulsed (6 ms) pulsed dye laser treatment of rosacea-associated telangiectasia using subpurpuric clinical threshold. *Dermatologic Surgery* **30**(1):37–40.

Katz B, Patel V (2006). Photodynamic therapy for the treatment of erythema, papules, pustules, and severe flushing consistent with rosacea. *Journal of Drugs in Dermatology* **5**(2 Suppl):6–8.

Kawana S, Ochiai H, Tachihara R (2007). Objective evaluation of the effect of intense pulsed light on rosacea and solar lentigines by spectrophotometric analysis of skin color. *Dermatologic Surgery* **33**(4):449–454.

Lonne-Rahm S, Nordlind K, Edstrom DW, Ros AM, Berg M (2004). Laser treatment of rosacea: a pathoetiological study. *Archives of Dermatology* **140**(11):1345–1349.

Lowe NJ, Behr KL, Fitzpatrick R, Goldman M, Ruiz-Esparza J (1991). Flash lamp pumped dye laser for rosacea-associated telangiectasia and erythema. *Journal of Dermatologic Surgery and Oncology* **17**(6):522–525.

Mark KA, Sparacio RM, Voigt A, Marenus K, Sarnoff DS (2003). Objective and quantitative improvement of rosacea-associated erythema after intense pulsed light treatment. *Dermatologic Surgery* **29**(6):600–604.

Nybaek H, Jemec GB (2005). Photodynamic therapy in the treatment of rosacea. *Dermatology* **211**(2):135–138.

Papageorgiou P, Clayton W, Norwood S, Chopra S, Rustin M (2008). Treatment of rosacea with intense pulsed light: significant improvement and long-lasting results. *British Journal of Dermatology* **159**(3):628–632.

Rohrer TE, Chatrath V, Iyengar V (2004). Does pulse stacking improve the results of treatment with variable-pulse pulsed-dye lasers? *Dermatologic Surgery* **30**(2 Pt 1):163–167.

Schroeter CA, Haaf-von Below S, Neumann HA (2005). Effective treatment of rosacea using intense pulsed light systems. *Dermatologic Surgery* **31**(10):1285–1289.

Sperber BR, Walling HW, Arpey CJ, Whitaker DC (2005). Vesiculobullous eruption from intense pulsed light treatment. *Dermatologic Surgery* **31**(3):345–348.

Tan SR, Tope WD (2004). Pulsed dye laser treatment of rosacea improves erythema, symptomatology, and quality of life. *Journal of the American Academy of Dermatology* **51**(4):592–599.

Tan ST, Bialostocki A, Armstrong JR (2004). Pulsed dye laser therapy for rosacea. *British Journal of Plastic Surgery* **57**(4):303–310.

Taub AF (2003). Treatment of rosacea with intense pulsed light. *Journal of Drugs in Dermatology* **2**(3):254–259.

Togsverd-Bo K, Wiegell SR, Wulf HC, Haedersdal M (2009). Short and limited effect of long-pulsed dye laser alone and in combination with photodynamic therapy for inflammatory rosacea. *Journal of the European Academy of Dermatology and Venereology* **23**(2):200–201.

Uebelhoer NS, Bogle MA, Stewart B, Arndt KA, Dover JS (2007). A split-face comparison study of pulsed 532 nm KTP laser and 595 pulsed dye laser in the treatment of facial telangiectasias and diffuse telangiectatic facial erythema. *Dermatologic Surgery* **33**(4):441–448.

West TB, Alster TS (1998). Comparison of the long-pulse dye (590–595 nm) and KTP (532 nm) lasers in the treatment of facial and leg telangiectasias. *Dermatologic Surgery* **24**(2):221–226.

Chapter 8

Aghassi D, Gonzalez E, Anderson RR, Rajadhyaksha M, Gonzalez S (2000). Elucidating the pulsed-dye laser treatment of sebaceous hyperplasia *in vivo* with real-time confocal scanning laser microscopy. *Journal of the American Academy of Dermatology* 43:49–53.

Akamatsu H, Zouboulis CC, Orfanos CE (1992). Control of human sebocyte proliferation *in vitro* by testosterone and 5-alpha-dihydrotestosterone is dependent on the localization of the sebaceous glands. *Journal of Investigative Dermatology* 99(4):509–511.

Alster TS, Tanzi EL (2003). Photodynamic therapy with topical aminolevulinic acid and pulsed dye laser irradiation for sebaceous hyperplasia. *Journal of Drugs in Dermatology* 2(5):501–504.

Bader RS, Scarborough DA (2000). Surgical pearl: intralesional electrodessication of sebaceous hyperplasia. *Journal of the American Academy of Dermatology* 42:127–128.

Boonchai W, Leenutaphong V (1997). Familial presenile sebaceous gland hyperplasia. *Journal of the American Academy of Dermatology* 36(1):120–122.

Burton CS, Sawchuk WS (1985). Premature sebaceous gland hyperplasia: successful treatment with isotretinoin. *Journal of the American Academy of Dermatology* 12:182–184.

De Berker DA, Taylor AE, Quinn AG, Simpson NB (1996). Sebaceous hyperplasia in organ transplant recipients: shared aspects of hyperplastic and dysplastic processes? *Journal of the American Academy of Dermatology* 35(5 Pt 1):696–699.

De Villez RL, Roberts LC (1982). Premature sebaceous gland hyperplasia. *Journal of the American Academy of Dermatology* 6(5):933–935.

Deplewski D, Rosenfield RL (2000). Role of hormones in pilosebaceous unit development. *Endocrine Reviews* 21(4):363–392.

Divaris DX, Kennedy JC, Pottier RH (1990). Phototoxic damage to sebaceous glands and hair follicles of mice after systemic administration of 5-aminolevulinic acid correlates with localized protoporphyrin IX fluorescence. *American Journal of Pathology* 136(4):891–897.

Dupre A, Bonafe JL, Lamon P (1983). Functional familial sebaceous hyperplasia of the face and premature sebaceous gland hyperplasia: a new and unique entity. *Journal of the American Academy of Dermatology* 9(5):768–769.

Ebling FJ (1957). The action of testosterone on the sebaceous glands and epidermis in castrated and hypophysectomized male rats. *Journal of Endocrinology* 15:297–306.

Ebling FJ (1967). The action of an antiandrogenic steroid, 17alpha-methyl-beta-nortestosterone, on sebum secretion in rats treated with testosterone. *Journal of Endocrinology* 38:181–185.

Epstein EH, Epstein WL (1966). New cell formation in human sebaceous glands. *Journal of Investigative Dermatology* 46:453–458.

Gold MH, Bradshaw VL, Boring MM, Bridges TM, Biron JA, Lewis TL (2004). Treatment of sebaceous gland hyperplasia by photodynamic therapy with 5-aminolevulinic acid and a blue light source or intense pulsed light source. *Journal of Drugs in Dermatology* 3(6 Suppl):S6–S9.

Goldman MP (2003). Using 5-aminolevulinic acid to treat acne and sebaceous hyperplasia. *Cosmetic Dermatology* 16:57–58.

Grekin RC, Ellis CN (1984). Isotretinoin for the treatment of sebaceous hyperplasia. *Cutis* 34:90–92.

Grimalt R, Ferrando J, Mascaro JM (1997). Premature familial sebaceous hyperplasia: successful response to oral isotretinoin in three patients. *Journal of the American Academy of Dermatology* 37(6):996–998.

Holbrook KA, Smith LT, Kaplan ED, Minami SA, Hebert GP, Underwood RA (1993). Expression of morphogens during human follicle development *in vivo* and a model for studying follicle morphogenesis *in vitro*. *Journal of Investigative Dermatology* 101(1 Suppl):39S–49S.

Hongcharu W, Taylor CR, Chang Y, Aghassi D, Suthamjariya K, Anderson RR (2000). Topical ALA-photodynamic therapy for the treatment of acne vulgaris. *Journal of Investigative Dermatology* 115(2):183–192.

Horio T, Horio O, Miyauchi-Hashimoto H, Ohnuki M, Isei T (2003). Photodynamic therapy of sebaceous hyperplasia with topical 5-aminolaevulinic acid and slide projector. *British Journal of Dermatology* 148(6):1274–1276.

Landthaler ML, Haina D, Waidelich W, Braun-Falco O (1984). A three-year experience with the argon laser in dermatotherapy. *Journal of Dermatologic Surgery and Oncology* 10:456–461.

Lesnik RH, Kligman LH, Kligman AM (1992). Agents that cause enlargement of sebaceous glands in hairless mice. II. Ultraviolet radiation. *Archives of Dermatological Research* 284(2):106–108.

No D, McClaren M, Chotzen V, Kilmer SL (2004). Sebaceous hyperplasia treated with a 1450 nm diode laser. *Dermatologic Surgery* 30(3):382–384.

Paithankar DY, Ross EV, Saleh BA, Blair MA, Graham BS (2002). Acne treatment with a 1,450 nm wavelength laser and cryogen spray cooling. *Lasers in Surgery and Medicine* 31(2):106–114.

Perrett CM, McGregor J, Barlow RJ, Karran P, Proby C, Harwood CA (2006). Topical photodynamic therapy with methyl aminolevulinate to treat sebaceous hyperplasia in an organ transplant recipient. *Archives of Dermatology* 142(6):781–782.

Plewig G, Christophers E, Braun-Falco O (1971). Cell transition in human sebaceous glands. *Acta Dermato-Venereologica* 51(6):423–428.

Pochi PE, Strauss JS, Downing DT (1979). Age-related changes in sebaceous gland activity. *Journal of Investigative Dermatology* 73(1):108–111.

Richey DF, Hopson B (2004). Treatment of sebaceous hyperplasia by photodynamic therapy. *Cosmetic Dermatology* 17:525–529.

Rosian R, Goslen JB, Brodell RT (1991). The treatment of benign sebaceous hyperplasia with the topical application of bichloracetic acid. *Journal of Dermatologic Surgery and Oncology* 17:876–879.

Salim A, Reece SM, Smith AG, et al. (2006). Sebaceous hyperplasia and skin cancer in patients undergoing renal transplant. *Journal of the American Academy of Dermatology* 55(5):878–881.

Sauter LS, Loud AV (1975). Morphometric evaluation of sebaceous gland volume in intact, castrated and testosterone treated rats. *Journal of Investigative Dermatology* 64:9–13.

Schonermark MP, Schmidt C, Raulin C (1997). Treatment of sebaceous gland hyperplasia with the pulsed dye laser. *Lasers in Surgery and Medicine* 21:313–316.

Schwartz RA, Torre DP (1995). The Muir–Torre syndrome: a 25-year retrospect. *Journal of the American Academy of Dermatology* 33(1):90–104.

Thody AJ, Shuster S (1989). Control and function of sebaceous glands. *Physiological Reviews* 69(2):383–416.

Thiboutot D, Sivarajah A, Gilliland K, Cong Z, Clawson G (2000). The melanocortin 5 receptor is expressed in human sebaceous glands and rat preputial cells. *Journal of Investigative Dermatology* 115(4):614–619.

Wheeland RG, Wiley MD (1987). Q-tip cryosurgery for the treatment of senile sebaceous hyperplasia. *Journal of Dermatologic Surgery and Oncology* 13:729–730.

Zouboulis CC, Bohm M (2004). Neuroendocrine regulation of sebocytes–a pathogenetic link between stress and acne. *Experimental Dermatology* 13(4 Suppl):31–35.

Zouboulis CC, Boschnakow A (2001). Chronological ageing and photoageing of the human sebaceous gland. *Clinical and Experimental Dermatology* 26(7):600–607.

Zouboulis CC, Seltmann H, Hiroi N, et al. (2002). Corticotropin-releasing hormone: an autocrine hormone that promotes lipogenesis in human sebocytes. *Proceedings of the National Academy of Sciences of the United States of America* 99(10):7148–7153.

Zouboulis CC, Xia L, Akamatsu H, et al. (1998). The human sebocyte culture model provides new insights into development and management of seborrhea and acne. *Dermatology* 196(1):21–31.

INDEX

Printed and bound by CPI Group (UK) Ltd, Croydon, CR0 4YY

23/10/2024

01778251-0016